Beyond Menopause

Beyond Menopause brings to light the unique healthcare needs of postmenopausal women. It offers women integrative-holistic approaches that bridge the gap between conventional medicine and systems of holistic healing. Integrative strategies are highlighted in the context of common health conditions, including anxiety, fatigue, sleep disturbance, sexual health, weight concerns, bone health, and brain health. Up-to-date information is provided about the use of hormone therapy during the menopause transition. Clinical vignettes illustrate how individual women explore pathways to better health through shared decision-making with their health practitioners.

Women of postmenopausal age want to remain healthy, vital, and engaged, yet they are often overlooked in the healthcare system. In this phase of life, women need to create their own integrative path to wellness. *Beyond Menopause* shows women how to prime their voice for self-advocacy and establish collaborative relationships with their health practitioners. Women are advised to create an adaptable network of practitioners to accommodate changing needs—their own "web of wellness."

Beyond Menopause brings a fresh perspective to the mental, physical, and spiritual elements of holistic living. From the distinct vantage points of medicine and neuroscience, the authors guide women toward new pathways to optimal health and well-being.

Beyond Menopause
New Pathways to Holistic Health

Carolyn Torkelson, MD
Catherine Marienau, PhD

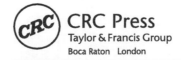

CRC Press
Taylor & Francis Group
Boca Raton   London

CRC Press is an imprint of the
Taylor & Francis Group, an **informa** business

First edition published 2023
by CRC Press
6000 Broken Sound Parkway NW, Suite 300, Boca Raton, FL 33487–2742

and by CRC Press
4 Park Square, Milton Park, Abingdon, Oxon, OX14 4RN

CRC Press is an imprint of Taylor & Francis Group, LLC

ISBN: 978-1-032-16916-3 (hbk)
ISBN: 978-1-032-16496-0 (pbk)
ISBN: 978-1-003-25096-8 (ebk)

DOI: 10.1201/9781003250968

Typeset in Times
by Apex CoVantage, LLC

For our daughters, Erica and Anna

Contents

PART III Harmonize Your Body, Mind, and Spirit

Foreword

A number of excellent books have been written about menopause, but few focus on the years beyond menopause, and very few offer a holistic approach. Carolyn Torkelson and Catherine Marienau are the perfect duo to write this book for women and health providers. Carolyn brings years of holistic clinical experience and research in women's health. Catherine brings years of experience as a mentor, teacher, and author in higher learning for women, and she co-hosts a weekly podcast featuring inspiring stories from women over 70. Their work with thousands of women over five decades is the cornerstone of this book. Their collaborative spirit creates a deeper and more inclusive perspective on women's holistic living.

Carolyn brings the same spirit to our collaboration as co-chairs of the Minnesota Holistic Medicine Group (MHMG), which I founded in the late 1980s. The MHMG is composed of 900 Minnesota healthcare practitioners from all disciplines. We connect with like-minded practitioners to learn from each other and support a referral network. The MHMG is a branch of our national organization, the Academy of Integrative Health and Medicine.

My path as an early adapter in holistic medicine began when my wife (a nurse) and I joined the Peace Corps in 1967. I was a medical doctor serving in Malaysia and Ghana, and part of my work was at an Aboriginal hospital near Kuala Lumpur. During those years, I was exposed to a wide range of healing modalities that expanded my vision and ideas of how healing can occur.

I returned to the United States to become one of the first physicians to complete a residency in family medicine. I found "my tribe" with the newly formed American Holistic Medical Association. Here were doctors who were interested not just in what was wrong with a patient but why the problem was occurring. I learned to always ask, "What is the body in its wisdom trying to tell this person?"

As integrative medicine moves to the forefront of heath care, I believe that everyone, after reading this book, will better understand the true meaning of holistic and integrated approaches to healthcare for postmenopausal women. The authors encourage women to know themselves and prime their voice for self-advocacy. The book goes beyond the physical aspects of the body by integrating emotional, social, spiritual, and environmental dimensions. Now that is holistic!

Congratulations to Carolyn and Catherine for this incredible book of information for every woman aged 40 and beyond.

Bill Manahan, MD
Assistant Professor Emeritus
University of Minnesota Medical School &
Academic Health Center
Academy of Integrative Health & Medicine,
Lee Lipsenthal Lifetime Achievement Award, 2016
Author of Eat for Health: Fast and Simple Ways of
Eliminating Diseases Without Medical Assistance

Preface

Ours is a friendship born out of a shared passion for adventure and wanting to make a difference in innovative ways. As young women born and raised in rural Minnesota, we lived relatively sheltered lives. Then, in the fall of 1967, college happened, and we left our small towns for university life. During the 1960s, college campuses were in turmoil with social justice issues including civil rights, student rights, women's rights, and the pervasive anti–Vietnam War movement. We studied hard and worked hard, and as graduation loomed on the horizon, the desire was brewing to explore and experience new adventures. So, the history major, Carolyn, and the anthropology major, Catherine, embarked on loosely planned, summer-long, independent study projects in Mexico.

Each equipped with a backpack, sleeping bag, two changes of clothes, and $200, we traveled third-class buses from West to East coasts with forays into southern and northern regions. We explored numerous archeological sites, from Teotihuacan to Palenque to Tulum. Too poor to hire a tour guide or even splurge on guidebooks, we nonetheless marveled at the sights, with admittedly limited understanding of what we were seeing.

The connection between this story and the story of how we came to write a book together, so many years later, lies in a little-known, enchanting island off the east coast of Mexico. In the summer of 1970, we hopped on a motorized rubber raft, leaving from a deserted white sand beach that thousands of tourists now know as Cancun, to arrive at Isla Mujeres—Island of Women. The native undeveloped beauty of the island inspired Carolyn (always the visionary) to pronounce "I will live here someday." Sure enough, more than 25 years ago, Carolyn and her husband purchased a condo on Isla Mujeres, and Catherine has been a regular wintertime visitor.

And so, our co-authorship was born. In February 2019, on Isla Mujeres, we spent a week sketching out an outline for *Beyond Menopause: New Pathways to Holistic Health*. We became excited about connecting our passions—integrative women's health and adult learning and the brain. We imagined that postmenopausal women—and their healthcare providers—could benefit from a focused look at common health conditions during this time of life and integrative approaches to address them. We imagined that women could become more engaged advocates and partners in their own healthcare.

Although we have been friends for more than 50 years, traveled and vacationed together, and talked extensively about our work in innovative education and health, *Beyond Menopause* is our first professional adventure as a duo. *Adventure* is the right word as we explored how to stay connected while living in different states (Illinois and Minnesota), express our collective and separate voices, identify the intersections of our expertise and perspectives, and present mature women as inspiring heroines through their stories of integrative health and well-being.

About the Authors

Carolyn Torkelson, MD

Dr. Torkelson's route from history major to integrative health physician has been circuitous. She began her health career as a nurse, eventually working as a nurse practitioner in a holistic clinic, an experience that inspired her to go to medical school with a focus on preventive care and holistic health. But once in practice, she quickly learned that Western medicine had few answers to the array of chronic illnesses that plagued her patients. She committed herself to find alternative solutions to the myriad problems and concerns she heard about every day. At the time, formal training programs in integrative-holistic medicine did not exist, so Dr. Torkelson studied botanical and functional medicine, explored self-care, and became active with the American Holistic Medical Association, a group of like-minded practitioners. What sets Dr. Torkelson apart is her quest to complement traditional medicine with her rich knowledge of other healing approaches. She spent a year in Guatemala working in a mission clinic, worked on the Turtle Mountain Indian Reservation in North Dakota, and spent time in northern India learning about Tibetan medicine.

After 10 years in family medicine, Dr. Torkelson joined the faculty of the University of Minnesota and completed a master's in clinical research. She has been involved in numerous research studies on integrative medicine. Since 2004, her clinical practice has focused on women's health and providing integrative healthcare to women of all ages. When she reflects on how she came to be an advocate for integrative healthcare, Dr. Torkelson realizes it was in incremental phases. In her words, "I did not have a transformative experience or an 'aha' moment that sent me on a quest for enlightenment. Rather, it was a slow emergence of an innate understanding that how we eat, think, sleep, and move affect our emotional and spiritual states." Dr. Torkelson is emblematic of many women her age who experience ups and downs, successes and failures, but more importantly, are infused with the desire to continue on a purposeful life journey.

Dr. Torkelson is on the boards of Pathways, a crisis healing center, and of the National BOlder Women's Health Coalition. She co-chairs the Minnesota Holistic Medicine Group, an organization that started 30 years ago and now connects 900 holistic providers from multiple healing disciplines. Although Dr. Torkelson retired from the University of Minnesota in December 2019, with the emergence of the coronavirus pandemic, she returned to a faculty position as a community preceptor.

Catherine Marienau, PhD

For more than 50 years, Dr. Marienau has been listening to women's stories in their pursuit of higher education. While serving as an academic tutor at the Center for Higher Education for Low-Income People (HELP) at the University of Minnesota, she witnessed the power of learning for nontraditional learners—people who because of age, location, life circumstance, or ethnic or racial identity—had been shut out of higher education. The women attending the HELP Center had especially inspiring life stories because they pursued learning in the face of enormous barriers, including limited finances, family responsibilities, work obligations, low self-esteem, unsupportive family and friends, and more.

Dr. Marienau continued serving adult learners in the University Without Walls program during its experimental start-up year in 1971, going on to become the program director and academic mentor from 1974 to 1983. Her philosophy was "the ethics of choice and care," and her goal was to reform higher education, along with providing access and quality learning opportunities for nontraditional or marginalized learners. Three-quarters of the students in the program were women in their 30s to 60s, a statistic that persists to this day in adult-focused programs across the country.

In 1983, Dr. Marienau joined the School for New Learning at DePaul University in Chicago, where, again, most learners were mature women. For 35 years, she taught a course on women's issues, in various formats. She conducted research on the barriers to higher education for rural women and on experiences of vital women in their 70s and beyond. Again, she based her mentoring on and practiced her philosophy of choice and care, working in partnership with women to ensure that their learning and its outcomes mattered.

Dr. Marienau holds a master's degree in the social and philosophic foundations of education, with an emphasis on anthropology and innovative higher education, and a doctorate in curriculum and instruction with an emphasis on adult higher education. She is a master practitioner of neuro-linguistic programming (NLP), which complements more recent study and writing in affective neuroscience and learning.

PERSONAL NOTES FROM THE AUTHORS

My inspiration to write about postmenopausal women comes directly from the many women I've seen and listened to throughout 30 years of clinical practice. Women have encouraged me to share their stories from a holistic perspective, one that touches on all aspects of well-being. Now, in the early phase of retirement from clinical practice, I am quieting my mind to recall their voices and listen to my inner voice, and to intertwine their stories and mine into a narrative that speaks to the heart of women. When Catherine agreed to co-author *Beyond Menopause*, I was excited (and relieved) that I could share thoughts, ideas, and stories with someone who has walked with me through the ups and downs of life for the last 50 years. It has been an honor to collaborate and write about women's journeys through the lens of innate learning and wisdom. Recently, I have developed a website (womenaginggwell.org) to provide women with holistic approaches and innovative pathways to optimize their health.

—Carolyn Torkelson, MD

In my doctoral studies, I was taught the prevailing models of human development that depicted women as less developed, intellectually and ethically, than men. Really? This is a prime example of reality disputing theory. I dedicated most of my career to mentoring women in their educational pursuits and supporting them in their quests for personal development. Since I turned 70 and retired from my full-time faculty position in 2019, I am fortunate to be collaborating with women colleagues on topics that matter to women. With them, I am extending my public voice: writing and consulting about neuroscience and adult learning; advocating for end-of-life options; contributing to a longitudinal study of vital women's experiences of aging; and co-hosting a podcast—*Women Over 70: Aging Reimagined*—that features women, ages 70 to 100+, who lead inspiring and meaningful lives (womenover70.com). The opportunity to co-author *Beyond Menopause* has added a whole new dimension to my mission to support aging women in creating their best life.

—Catherine Marienau, PhD

Introduction: Women Coming of Age

If you are a woman beyond menopause, you likely have one-third or more of your life left to live. You are part of the growing female demographic—older women who have unique healthcare needs yet are subject to a health system that has both historically and currently overlooked them. Rather than settle for being ignored, we believe that women can learn to advocate more forcefully for the care they need. With 30–50 years left to live after menopause, we want you to optimize your health no matter where you are on the health spectrum. We believe that women benefit most from a preventive and integrative approach to health that addresses their diverse needs.

Postmenopausal women are growing in numbers. The baby boomers, born between 1946 and 1964, make up a large portion of postmenopausal women and are living long, healthy lives. Members of the Silent Generation and Generation X are also part of this growing demographic. American women aged 65 and older tripled between 2005 and 2015 and will double again by 2030.[1] This unprecedented number of women presents the healthcare system with significant healthcare challenges and many opportunities for improvement. We are at the precipice of transformative change! We need a more comprehensive, integrative healthcare system that reaches beyond the conventional model and considers other wellness systems and healing modalities. Leading this charge are older women who have matured through decades of paternalistic socialization about health, as well as gender, race, and age discrimination.

THE MYTHS OF SEXISM AND AGEISM

Consider the environment in which most contemporary postmenopausal women were raised. *Sexism,* a term first introduced in 1968, was embedded in societal messages that permeated our lives. The roles for many of our mothers were well defined: a domestic life centered on childbearing and childrearing, homemaking, and being a good wife. Many of us growing up in the '50s and '60s faced limited choices and opportunities, just because of our gender. For example, in most schools, formalized sports activities were available only for boys, so exercise did not become a regular part of girls' lives. On the career front, young women were encouraged to consider chiefly secretarial, nursing, or teaching roles. These discriminatory limitations placed on girls and women fit comfortably into daily life without much thought.

Many of us came of age in the 1960s when social turmoil, women's and civil rights movements, and educational innovations were exposing the many discriminations faced by women. Despite the pressures to comply with social norms and sexism, the postmenopausal women of today have been trailblazers in every phase of their adult lives. We have integrated higher education; entered and changed the workforce; and redefined sexuality, marriage, childbearing, and parenting.

As we get older, ageism becomes another layer of disregard that profoundly affects our lives. The term *ageism,* first coined in 1969, is defined as "a process of systematic stereotyping and discrimination against people because they are old."[2] Or, consider Margaret Gullette's contemporary take on ageism as "the affliction of suffering by mere fact of birthdate."[3] We are dispelling the sexist beliefs that gender limits us and that women's actions and influences are less powerful than those of men. We wholly reject the cultural belief that aging and older women serve no purpose. Women with many years to live beyond menopause are claiming purpose, passion, and joy that can and does have profound influence on themselves, the community, and the generations to come. We are the mature women with the knowledge, wisdom, experience, and stories to share with younger generations.

Women who are now in their postmenopausal years have led diverse lives and faced unprecedented challenges and opportunities. We do not tie our identity to chronological age, yet we are, indeed, aging, which brings with it particular healthcare needs. Although most of us have had considerable experience with healthcare, for both ourselves and our families, the postmenopausal time is relatively unexplored territory. Learning how to proactively communicate for attention and dignity in healthcare can help you mitigate the frustration that commonly accompanies aging. We are encouraged by emerging age-friendly trends in communities, services, and structures that encourage active aging.

ADVOCACY FOR HEALTHCARE

In efforts to reshape the healthcare frontier, we ask, *how can we become our own advocates in a healthcare system that currently does not meet the needs of aging women*? The healthcare system of today focuses almost exclusively on the diagnosis and treatment of acute and chronic disease rather than on promotion of wellness. Certainly, we recognize the value of serving patients in times of illness and in national crises, such as the coronavirus pandemic. We are not asking for the conventional healthcare system to abandon its previously excellent efforts. However, we do expect healthcare to be inclusive of other healing systems and options for care. Women are frustrated with the limited time they have with their physician and the technology that distances them from their healthcare team. For these and other reasons, confidence in our health system has eroded. It's time for women to take action.

As advocates for optimal health of aging women, our stance is that healthcare must shift from the disease-centric approach to incorporating scientific wellness components, such as nutrition, physical exercise, and mind-body practices, along with guidance from traditional health systems to promote wellness. We invite healthcare practitioners to develop a partnership with their patients and to foster a comprehensive, integrative approach to care in ways that value each woman's story.

Beyond Menopause is for women who want to exercise their voice, engage in holistic-integrative approaches, and participate in their healthcare in partnership with their health providers. It is for women who want the most progressive approach to living fully and staying physically, mentally, and spiritually healthy.

Now is the time for women to become their own advocates and claim the kind of healthcare they deserve to live well. We urge women to know their whole selves as they strive to live their best life, regardless of age or life story.

GETTING THE MOST OUT OF *BEYOND MENOPAUSE*

We suggest beginning *Beyond Menopause* by reading the chapters in Part I because they provide an informative and rich context for the rest of the book. The chapters in Part II, which focus on specific health conditions, can be read in any sequence according to your interests. Part III can be read whenever the spirit moves you, although waiting until the end might have the most impact. We hope you will read parts of this book many times over as you develop an emboldened approach to your health and well-being.

Please note that as co-authors, we speak as "we" when the content and structure of the text represent our collaborative decisions. However, Part II (Chapters 4–11) of *Beyond Menopause* includes a number of women's stories from Carolyn's clinical practice, so you will hear her speak as "I" in the first-person singular voice. On occasion, Carolyn also offers her particular medical views and those, too, are relayed in her first-person voice.

Part I

Speak Up for Yourself

In Chapters 1 through 3, we introduce you to the principles of holistic and integrative health, followed by two crucial, yet often overlooked, aspects of well-being: self-advocating for your own health and building supportive relationships with your health providers. Postmenopausal women need to be able to advocate for their needs with all their healthcare practitioners. You can create your own web of wellness that is guided by an integrative model of health and healing. You know best what you need to live a full and vital life, and you possess the agency to ask for it.

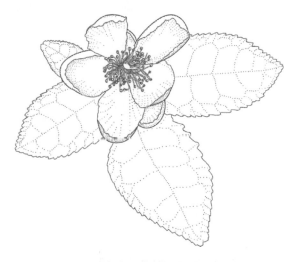

Camellia sinensis (Green Tea)

DOI: 10.1201/9781003250968-1

Part I

Speak Up for Yourself

1 Elements of Holistic Integrative Health

You are a woman of postmenopausal age or soon to become one. How would you characterize your health right now? Perhaps you feel well enough, yet would like to feel more vigorous overall. Or maybe you are dealing with a bothersome condition that just isn't resolving. Or more alarmingly, maybe something major is going on that needs serious attention.

Whatever your situation, if you're reading this book, you're likely looking to optimize your health. You may have found that conventional healthcare does not adequately address the range and types of conditions you are experiencing. You are not alone. Many postmenopausal women want comprehensive healing approaches that include nonconventional care. But where do you look for alternatives? What can you expect? Whom do you trust? And, most importantly, why even go down that path?

We believe holistic integrative health is a perfect platform for you to receive the best of both conventional and nonconventional care. *Beyond Menopause* is intended to help you bridge the gap between the two so you can optimize your health and well-being, no matter where you are on the health spectrum.

MANY TERMS, MANY PERSPECTIVES

Integrative medicine, also referred to as integrative health, encompasses and embraces diverse perspectives and disciplines within the healing field of healthcare. Different organizations and practitioners offer somewhat different definitions.

INTEGRATIVE MEDICINE

Integrative medicine and health reaffirms the importance of the relationship between practitioner and patient, focuses on the whole person, is informed by evidence, and makes use of all appropriate therapeutic and lifestyle approaches, healthcare professionals, and disciplines to achieve optimal health and healing.

Academic Consortium for Integrative Medicine & Health

Integrative medicine is a type of medical care that combines conventional (standard) medical treatment with complementary and alternative (CAM) therapies that have been shown to be safe and to work. CAM therapies treat the mind, body, and spirit.

National Cancer Institute

We have constructed this definition: Integrative health is a philosophy of living one's life from a holistic perspective. It is a healing approach to medicine that attends to the whole person—body, mind, and spirit—by combining conventional medicine with other traditions of health systems and healing modalities. It addresses the fundamentals of lifestyle and self-care and emphasizes a therapeutic relationship between patient and practitioner to create wellness.

As the field of integrative medicine has matured, a plethora of terms have evolved, including holistic medicine, alternative medicine, complementary alternative medicine, mind-body medicine, blended medicine, functional medicine, restorative medicine, root-cause medicine, transformative health care, personalized medicine, and precision medicine. No matter what label is placed on this style of medicine, we think it is best described by the word *holistic* and speaks to how we want to approach women's health and healing.

For many patients and practitioners, a gap exists between conventional medicine and other healing systems and modalities (historically referred to as alternatives). Sometimes, the gap can seem more like a chasm, but it need not be. An important role of integrative medicine is to serve as a bridge between conventional and nonconventional approaches.

Central to the healing process is the need for the healthcare system to support wellness. We all hear it every day: "Our healthcare system is a mess." The United States has excellent physicians, nurses, and many other dedicated providers, so what's getting in the way of providing the care women want? While the reasons are numerous and complex, the crux of the problem is that our healthcare system focuses almost exclusively on the diagnosis and treatment of disease rather than on the promotion of wellness. Improvement will require system-level change, shifting from a disease-centric approach to one that incorporates a scientific wellness component. We need restructured care models and teams that use nutrition, physical exercise, and mind-body practices, along with guidance from traditional health systems, to promote wellness and healing.[1] This inclusive model represents a whole system of healing that is the cornerstone of integrative medicine.

Integrative medicine provides a compass for individualized care within a broad array of options for better health. Our experience underscores three principles of integrative medicine that are especially appealing to women: the whole-systems approach, the healing power of love, and the patient-practitioner partnership.

The Whole-Systems Approach: The core principle of integrative medicine is a whole-systems approach that involves a conscious pursuit of the highest level of physical, mental, emotional, and spiritual well-being. Your body has the inherent ability to establish, maintain, and restore health. The role of the integrative practitioner is to facilitate and augment this process, to identify and remove obstacles to health and recovery. A whole-systems approach considers your relationships, as well as the social influences and environmental factors that impact your everyday life and overall health. It offers a range of healing strategies that will engage you in new pathways to better health.

The Healing Power of Love: The second principle concerns a powerful, sometimes taken for granted, ingredient: the healing power of love. Holistic integrative practitioners strive to relate to patients with grace, kindness, and acceptance. The essence of unconditional love starts with your own self-love and self-acceptance of who you are—just as you are. Unconditional love is about self-care and having compassion for yourself in all kinds of situations. It is the foundation of healing.

The Patient-Practitioner Partnership: The third principle is that patient and practitioner are in a partnership relationship in the healing process. You participate fully in the creation, advocacy, and coordination of your treatment plan. Your practitioner's aim is to personalize your care so that strategies for health improvement, and sticking to those strategies, can meet your unique lifestyle needs and challenges. We use the term *practitioners* because the spectrum of care you need may require an interdisciplinary approach that will involve different kinds of practitioners from the healing community. This is what we refer to as your *web of wellness*. Always keep in mind that your web of wellness is unique to you.

The following letter from one of Carolyn's patients illustrates the value of you and your practitioner working together as partners in your care.

Dear Dr. Torkelson,

I wanted to share with you that about a month ago, I dreamed that you called me just to tell me how glad you were that I was doing so well (I am!). I remembered that you, too, had to work at times to stay in touch with your joy, and that you hoped I was taking advantage of this opportunity to get in touch with mine. This dream has had such a profound effect on me, and so I wanted to share it. I often ask myself if I am "taking this opportunity" and will often just meditate on "my joy." I don't know how you manage to pull off this kind of "house call," but wow! I can't tell you what it means to have the type of doctor-patient relationship when you can be symbolic of my inner physician. Thank you for the good care you provide me.

WOMEN'S HEALTH GOALS

The demand for integrative practitioners and integrative care is growing. It is women like yourself who are the driving force behind this movement, who are willing to step outside the confines of traditional medicine to help themselves and their families stay well.

In 2012, a qualitative research project conducted by the School of Nursing in collaboration with the Women's Health Clinic (University of Minnesota) examined the needs of the mature woman from an integrative perspective. Four strong themes emerged from what these women reported as their goals for health care:

- Access to holistic integrative/alternative care
- A partnership relationship with their primary provider
- Wellness balance in their life for optimal health
- Achievable goals and strategies for healthy living as they age

Most likely, you can relate to one or more of these goals. Perhaps we should call them aspirations, because they are challenging to achieve if your conventional practitioner is not knowledgeable about other systems of health and other modalities of healing. If that is the case with your primary provider, at least you would want her to be open to, rather than critical or dismissive of, the choices you make regarding alternative options. Otherwise, like Mary, you may be in for some frustrating experiences.

> *Mary frequently sees her alternative practitioner for muscle testing to determine what herbs, supplements, or medications are safe for her to take. Mary believes muscle testing is a way that her body signals if the medication prescribed is "right" for her. When Mary's conventional doctor wants to prescribe a new medication, Mary asks if she can have one pill to take to her practitioner for testing before she starts taking the medication. Her doctor doesn't know what Mary is talking about when it comes to muscle testing and, being skeptical about this approach, dismisses her request. Mary becomes angry and frustrated with the doctor for not understanding and respecting the integrative approach she believes works best for her.*

An integrative care physician might explain to Mary that expecting her conventional doctor to understand and endorse her integrative plan would be ideal but is unrealistic. Although Mary would like all her practitioners to be on the same page with her, she needs to understand that each practitioner views her care through their particular lens of expertise and experience.

Fortunately, conventional practitioners coming out of training these days are showing more interest in and respect for other systems of healing. They have grown up around alternative practices that have been increasingly incorporated into daily living over the last 30 years. The use of chiropractors, osteopaths, acupuncturists, and naturopaths is becoming more mainstream. Conventional practitioners are also increasingly aware that people in different cultures want to incorporate their own Indigenous healers and traditions.

PILLARS OF HEALTH

From the holistic health perspective, your body is designed to heal. Engaging in the five pillars of health is the foundation for healing and optimizing your health. Let's look at each pillar individually.

> #1: *Restoration and sleep* help replenish and balance your energy. Getting 7–8 hours of restful sleep every night is primary. Beyond sleep, other restorative practices signal the body to find its inner calm. The goal of restoration is to nurture your body to do what it knows how to do—to heal.
>
> #2: *Nutrition and digestion* feed your gut-brain health. Eating whole foods is the best way to improve health and prevent disease. Good nutrition stabilizes metabolic function, reduces inflammation, and supports the immune system. Food is medicine, and its goal is to feed your body and mind.
>
> #3: *Movement and exercise* feed your body-brain health. Exercise and movement are powerful tools to increase your energy flow, improve your balance, support your bones, and maintain good posture. Movement stimulates your brain in ways that can enhance your thinking, relationships, and sense of well-being. The goal of movement is to nurture your vitality and self-confidence.

#4: *Emotional well-being* centers on nurturing your emotional and mental health. It involves having an awareness of your feelings and emotions, as well as the ability to appropriately manage and express them. A positive sense of well-being enables you to function in society and meet the demands of everyday life. The goal of emotional well-being is to nurture your resilience and sense of purpose.

#5: *Connection* empowers your social self. As relational beings, women especially value friendships. It is in community where you can know yourself more fully, extend care and kindness to others, and foster your curiosity outside of yourself. The goal of connection is to nurture your sense of belonging.

While we talk about these pillars independently and you might attend to one over the other, the pillars are actually highly interdependent. As you engage in one pillar, often the other pillars become healthier. When you strengthen your body, mind, and spirit connection, your overall health improves.

In an integrative model of care, you, as the patient, are always at the center. As you learn more about yourself and your unique needs, you can become more adept at knowing when and why to use the integrative tools available to you. Orchestrating your own care almost always involves advocating for what you want. We believe this role is so important that we devote the next chapter to self-advocacy.

2 Your Voice of Self-Advocacy

Here you are, in the last decades of your life, with more opportunities than ever to embrace holistic care of your body, mind, and spirit. To take advantage of these opportunities, you will need to develop and assert your voice of self-advocacy, both within yourself and with your health providers. Now is the time to advocate for your health and well-being!

You might be the woman who sits quietly waiting for your physician to ask questions and give direction. Or you might come to your physician knowing what you want, armed with a list of questions and requests. Or maybe you have already branched out beyond conventional medicine and need to educate your physician about interdisciplinary, holistic approaches that could improve your quality of life.

PRIMING YOUR VOICE

No matter where you are now on the advocacy continuum, you can prime your voice to advocate for what you need. How well do you know yourself in this regard? We get it—few of us were born with the self-advocacy gene, especially when it comes to navigating the healthcare system. You may shy away from it, feeling uneasy about speaking up. Or maybe you have already developed a high comfort level with self-advocacy. In any case, understanding how your brain works should help you develop your vocal priming powers.

The Anxious Brain and the Curious Brain: At its most basic level, your brain is playing a game of tug-of-war. Your anxious brain directs you to move *away* from something it perceives as negative or taxing, while your curious brain directs you to move *toward* something it perceives as positive or rewarding. Your anxious brain is likely to go on high alert when you encounter unknowns in the medical arena. Wanting to keep you safe, your brain's survival impulses kick in to help you deal with the situation. You'll feel as if you want to flee or shut down, stick with what you already know, rush to a decision, or make up a comforting story. These protective impulses, while natural, can inhibit your ability to advocate for yourself.

Margaret's story illustrates how the anxious brain versus the curious brain can play out in real life.

> *At age 72, Margaret has a series of major health problems that have resulted in anxiety and depression. She manages quite well with an antidepressant medication, but after returning from a short trip and realizing she cannot find her last 30-day supply of her prescription, Margaret's anxious thoughts are triggered: "I can't call and ask my doctor for a refill. She'll think I'm incompetent or, even worse, that I'm abusing the medication." Margaret asks her pharmacy for a refill, but her request is declined without the doctor's authorization for a new prescription. Margaret feels embarrassed*

DOI: 10.1201/9781003250968-3

Anxious Brain	Curious Brain
Reacts now	Invites new information
Feels afraid, nervous, uneasy	Wants to know the "why"
Knows and is right	Seeks alternative options
Takes short cuts	Takes time to reflect

Source: Adapted from Taylor K, Marienau C. *Facilitating Learning with the Adult Brain in Mind: A Conceptual and Practical Guide.* Jossey-Bass, Inc.; 2016.

and at fault for losing the medication. She decides she can manage, even though her anxiety symptoms are beginning to flare up. Margaret just cannot bring herself to contact her doctor, given her assumptions and fears. She finally confides her worries to a friend, who strongly urges Margaret to contact her physician. Only with this support does Margaret contact her physician, who approves the refill without hesitation or judgment.

How could the story be different if Margaret called on her curious brain to advocate for the assistance she needs?

As soon as Margaret realizes she misplaced the last 30 days of her antidepressant medication, she calls her pharmacy to explain the situation and request a refill. Her request is denied, and she is told she must either wait a month for a refill or obtain a new prescription. Knowing she cannot go a month without her medication, Margaret calls her doctor's office. The nurse promises a same day callback, but 2 days later, Margaret still has not heard from her doctor's office and no prescription refill has been called in to the pharmacy. Margaret again contacts her doctor's office, insisting on a callback that day, which she receives. Her doctor refills the medication and assures Margaret that her persistence in getting her medication refilled was the right approach.

In these two scenarios, Margaret's anxious brain is fearful and avoids dealing directly with the problem, while her curious brain wonders how best to solve the problem. When Margaret's curious brain is in charge, she can think proactively rather than reactively. She can determine that the benefit of refilling her prescription far outweighs the risk of her doctor's possible negative judgments.

To best advocate for your needs, you need to be aware of how your propensity for feeling anxious or curious influences how you think and act. How you come to know yourself is a complex matter, because your conscious mind is the last to know what's going on. Before coming into your conscious mind, emotions are already germinating in your somatic mind, that is, in your body. Body-based emotions carry very important messages, but you need to know how to listen and take time to do so.

WAYS OF KNOWING

Let's look at the different ways of knowing yourself, which are key to priming your voice for self-advocacy. First, we'll explore ways of knowing that arise from the unconscious realm: emotion and intuition. Next, we'll turn to conscious knowing—the cognitive domain, where we'll examine different perspectives on ways of knowing and their implications for developing your self-advocacy voice.

EMOTION

Only a century or so ago, the medical profession classified menopause as a physical disease that diminished a woman's intellectual ability and escalated her emotional state. Women's emotions and independent acts were actually diagnosed as hysterical. Historically, medical science has been so wary of women's emotions that many of us were taught to tamp down our emotions when interacting with medical personnel lest we be judged out of control or, worse, out of our minds.

Yet, it is a fact that your emotions are powerful influencers on your thoughts and actions. Are you aware that your emotions actually *live in* your body?[1] Emotions can control your body state, such as a feeling in the pit of your stomach, a fullness in your throat, or a flutter in your heart. Such sensations alert you when you feel threatened, such as by a health situation, and you feel confused, afraid, or frustrated. On the other hand, that sensation in your stomach, throat, or heart could be a signal of positive emotion when you received good test results or hear about a promising alternative. You might be feeling curiosity, excitement, or hope. According to Eckhart Tolle, author and spiritual teacher, your emotion arises at the place where mind and body meet. It is the body's reaction to your mind—a reflection of your mind in the body.[2]

Knowing yourself involves listening to your body. You probably agree that it's desirable to be aware of your emotions and how they manifest in your body. Unfortunately, many of us have been taught to tune out signals from our bodies and can even become alienated from them. More than 400 years ago, the philosopher Descartes warned against listening to the body because the senses are too easily deceived. Even though Descartes was proved wrong, day-to-day busyness might hamper you from noticing body signals that you are tired, off-kilter, or unfocused. You might be preoccupied by inner chatter, which can be distracting, especially if your inner critic is talking loudly.

Catherine's story (co-author) illustrates how emotions and external circumstances can interfere with listening to and learning from your body.

I have dealt with chronic, sometimes acute, lower back and upper leg pain for 35 years. Intermittently, I have used pain medications and steroid injections along with alternative modalities such as naprapathy, Feldenkrais, acupuncture, therapeutic exercise, and chiropractic. I was managing relatively well with acupuncture, regular exercise, and working with a personal trainer, until emotional stresses—preparing to leave full-time work (after nearly 50 years), celebrating my 70th birthday and retirement with travel and parties, and starting major new projects—took a toll. When my radiating back pain flared, I took more ibuprofen, continued with acupuncture, and added chiropractic treatments. I noticed, but ignored, blisters on my inner thigh. In spite of experiencing searing, unrelenting pain that left me unable to sleep for more than 2 hours at a stretch, I just kept on going. A friend finally insisted that I see my primary care doctor, whom I had been avoiding believing that the only thing that conventional medicine had to offer was pain medication, which would cause fuzzy thinking and interfere with my writing projects. To my surprise, I was diagnosed with shingles and post-herpetic neuralgia and needed treatment with prednisone and gabapentin. I was shocked to learn that the shingles vaccine I'd received 3 years ago, which I assumed protected me, was only 50% effective. The shingles pain subsided in my left thigh. For some months to come, I continued on gabapentin, saw my chiropractor three times a week, and made weekly visits to my acupuncturist and personal trainer. Over time, my back condition returned to a manageable state.

The survival impulses of Catherine's brain were clearly activated. She was stuck in what she already knew about how to treat her chronic back condition. She ignored the signals that the pain in her left thigh was a new pain, unlike her previous experiences. The severe pain and lack of sleep disrupted her ability to think clearly and to recognize that something very unusual was going on. Her emotions were in turmoil while trying to carry out huge responsibilities during a time of major life transition. Her anxious brain was doing its best to protect her, unfortunately, by avoiding high alerts from her body.

Without being fully conscious of it, Catherine was suppressing her emotions and operating as though she could control "mind over body." And because Catherine was masterful at masking her discomforts, most people saw her as managing very well. She was missing the whole picture, and it took a close friend to mobilize her to do something different. Had Catherine listened to her body and been seen by her physician earlier, she could have minimized the length of her illness and severity of suffering.

Both Margaret's and Catherine's stories reflect strong, complex emotions. In a health situation, your body-based emotions are cues for what to pay attention to. Listening to them is the first step, and somatic therapies can help you do just that. Somatic approaches (*soma,* from the early Greek, refers to the living body in its wholeness) can be very effective. A variety of techniques, including relaxation, breathwork, and meditation, involve a natural feedback loop between your body's sensations and your mind's thoughts. Living in your body, being awake and aware of your emotions and how they affect you, is a powerful form of knowing the essence of who you are. This awareness evokes greater self-confidence and self-compassion. Knowing yourself is a fundamental source of your own healing.

INTUITION

Emotion drives your responses toward or away from something. Intuition enables you to interpret the direction you are heading and give it meaning. Imagine a space in your body that holds what you don't know but could. Intuition bridges the gap between the conscious and unconscious parts of your mind. It is the ability to know something directly, without needing to impose logical reasoning or understand how you know it. Sometimes referred to as the "sixth sense" or "third eye," intuition is more than a psychic flash or reflexive emotional response. Intuition is like a compass that directs you to a place of deep knowing, an inclination you really can't explain but seems trustworthy.

In *Women's Intuition*, Paula Reeves describes intuition as a nonverbal, innate body wisdom that each of us has the capacity to know.[3] In Carolyn's practice, she has heard many women talk about the deep sense of knowing that guides them. They describe this knowing as an energy or vibration, a muse or messenger, or even information from a higher power or spiritual connection.

Strong expressions of intuition can guide you beyond what your intellect can know, and women are often credited with having intuitive powers. One explanation, in scientific terms, is found in anatomy. Women have a wider corpus callosum, which is the connective tissue that serves as the pathway between the left and right hemispheres of the brain. Women potentially have easier access to the emotional and intuitive knowing of the right hemisphere than men do. We can tamp down the logical left hemisphere that wants to challenge or invalidate our intuitions. Advances in the science of psychoneuroimmunology help us understand that body wisdom is transmitted through neurotransmitters, hormones, breath, heartbeat, and touch. Thus, we use intuition to tap into and read those body signals.

Intuition communicates through our bodies, sending subtle signals that are experienced through images, senses, dreams, messages, and symbols. Several different techniques can help you tap into your intuition. For example, guided imagery can help you visualize a journey deep within yourself. Movement or dance often evokes a natural emergence of the creative self. Journaling dreams, thoughts, and ideas also can evoke intuition, especially when you free-write without editing or censoring yourself. Similarly, attention to your kinesthetic senses—touch, smell, or hearing—can induce a deeper state of knowing.

We encourage you to let your intuition percolate and then trust the potent messages that emerge. Intuition is a skill to be sharpened. It is an essential resource for developing your self-advocacy voice on the path to well-being.

Cognitive Perspectives

After decades of human development theories and models telling women that we are less well developed than men (based on studies of young white males), four female researchers turned the tables. In their study of women of diverse ages and social circumstances, they revealed five ways of knowing, which they refer to as perspectives: (1) silent, (2) received, (3) subjective, (4) procedural, and (5) constructed.[4] You may have already developed the full repertoire of perspectives or maybe tend to rely on just a few. We invite you to consider how these perspectives can affect the potency of your advocacy voice.

The five major cognitive perspectives on ways of knowing—*silent, received, subjective, procedural*, and *constructed*—are not intended to be used as labels or to suggest that you are just one kind of knower. In the changing context of your healthcare, you might identify with a particular way of knowing at different times. We encourage you to pay attention to which perspectives under what circumstances might be an asset or a limitation. Reading the following details and stories of women who have been faced with major health decisions may help you develop and assert your advocacy voice.

Women's Ways of Knowing

Perspective	Characteristics
Silent knowers	Don't know how to begin to acquire knowledge
	Don't believe they can know things on their own
Received knowers	Can think for themselves but are uncomfortable with ambiguity
	Depend on external voices of authorities (eg, doctors) to influence their opinions, decisions, and actions
Subjective knowers	Rely on personal experience as the basis for what they know
	Hold strong conviction that what they already know is correct, often influenced by those people closest to them
Procedural knowers	Recognize that multiple perspectives exist
	Can exercise the voice of reason, but do so in two distinct ways from quite different starting points
Separate knowers	Enter an experience or situation with a "doubting voice"
	Look for what is flawed, incomplete, or unsubstantiated
	Reason with a debate style, favoring logic and critical analysis
Connected knowers	Enter an experience or a situation with a "believing voice"
	Look for what they can appreciate and understand of the other person's point of view
	Reason through empathy, connection, and careful listening
Constructed knowers	Integrate their received, subjective, and procedural knowing abilities to form their own base of knowing, with careful analysis and with empathic responses
	Have personal agency and can adapt to changes in their lives

Source: Adapted from Belenky MF, Clinchy BM, Goldberger NR, et al. *Women's Ways of Knowing: The Development of Self, Voice, and Mind.* Basic Books; 1996.

DEVELOPING YOUR VOICE

SILENT, RECEIVED, AND SUBJECTIVE KNOWERS

The most passive voice is *silent*, meaning that you literally have no voice to express yourself. Most of you will not identify with being a *silent knower*. However, it is not unusual to be thrown into this state when faced with disturbing, unanticipated news. For example, being told that your breast biopsy revealed cancer—even though the surgeon had assured you this would not be the case—can numb your senses. For a time, you may feel silenced, not knowing what or even how to think.

If you have dealt with a difficult health situation that is new or has serious implications, you may be familiar with the still relatively passive voice of a *received knower*. While you can think for yourself, you feel uncomfortable with not knowing enough. You hear what the options are but interpreting them is quite another matter. You look to the doctor, the external authority, as your primary source for knowing. In her clinical practice, Carolyn often hears: "I've been thinking about the options you say are available to me, but I'd like to follow your advice on what to do."

If you are a *subjective knower*, you assume a more active voice. Your main source of knowing is yourself or the people closest to you. You are not easily swayed by views or opinions from outside your trusted circle.

> *Maria complained to her physician of escalating worry over three significant stressors in her life: possible job loss, her husband's illness, and her daughter's pending divorce. When her doctor advised taking antianxiety medication, Maria responded emphatically, "No, I would never take medication. My best friend became suicidal on a drug like that. I will just continue with my daily meditation practice and will be fine with that."*

When you operate from *silent* or *received knowing* perspectives, you are influenced most by external authorities. When you operate from a *subjective knowing* perspective, you trust your intuitions and listen to your own voice over those of authorities or experts. Your self-advocacy voice is emerging, but you are not yet well equipped to exercise self-advocacy that is reasoned.

ASSERTING YOUR VOICE

PROCEDURAL KNOWERS

Advocating for yourself needs your voice of reason, seen in *procedural knowing*. Having been a consumer of knowledge and conventional healthcare for much of your life, you likely are familiar with reasoning being associated with critical thinking and skepticism. This *separate knowing* is a kind of "prove it to me" stance. The *women's ways of knowing* researchers discovered another kind of reasoning that favors appreciative thinking and acceptance (remember, these were all women). This *connected knowing* stance is: *"I want to understand what you mean."*

Again, there are two types of procedural knowers—*separate knowers* and *connected knowers*—that represent very different starting points.

As a *separate knower*, you bring your capacities for logical thinking and critical analysis to the health situation. Your "doubting voice" quickly alerts you to information that is incomplete or opinion that is unsubstantiated. For example, Lydia was considering taking hormone therapy for hot flashes that were disrupting her daily activity and sleep.

> *I have read the latest articles on the Women's Health Initiative. The study reports that breast cancer risk is low in the first 3–5 years of hormone therapy. However, a recent meta-analysis on hormone therapy indicates a greater risk of breast cancer than what is reported in the Women's Health Initiative study. I am a critical thinker and need more convincing evidence before starting on hormone therapy.*

Another patient, Lorna, had osteoporosis and anticipated a hip fracture if she were to fall.

> *My mother fell and broke her hip and never really recovered after surgery. My endocrinologist has strongly advised that I go on medication to prevent further bone loss. I have reviewed the literature on the medication and there are some bad side effects, like atypical fracture of the femur and jaw necrosis. Although these bad side effects are reported as rare, I remain unwilling to risk taking this medication.*

The "believing voice" of *connected knowers* sounds quite different. You are attuned to what you can appreciate and understand of another's point of view. Your reasoning process centers on careful listening to what you hear, read, and talk about. Cynthia, like Lorna, had osteoporosis and knew a fall could result in a hip fracture.

> *My mother fell and broke her hip and never really recovered after surgery. My endo-crinologist has strongly advised that I go on medication to prevent further bone loss. I have reviewed the literature on the medication, and there are some bad side effects. But if you look at the statistics, these side effects are rare. I have spoken to two other women in situations like mine, and I listened at length about their decision to start medication. I need lots of dialogue before I can make the right decision for myself.*

Another connected knower perspective is represented by Gretchen, who weighed the benefits of hormone therapy against the risk of breast cancer.

> *I have consulted with Dr. Torkelson and read the latest studies from the North American Menopause Society. I believe that hormone therapy would help me feel bet-ter and that the risk is low, but I am still conflicted about starting medication, even if I keep having yearly mammograms. I need to talk through the decision a bit more and hear about what other women have done in my situation. I'm curious as to what you would do, Dr. Torkelson, if you were in my shoes?*

These women are all procedural knowers who are engaged in valid reasoning pro-cesses. Lydia and Lorna illustrate a separate knowing perspective, whereas Cynthia and Gretchen proceed from a connected knowing perspective. From different start-ing points, they each arrived at what, for them, were sound decisions.

CONSTRUCTED KNOWERS

During the postmenopausal decades, women's health conditions can become more complex and carry heavy emotional weight. Wouldn't it be grand if all of us could function from a *constructed knowing* perspective? Essentially, this means that you would be able to integrate all three knowing abilities (received, subjective, procedural) into your advocacy voice. You can consider things both critically and appreciatively. You are willing and able to question your own thoughts and assumptions. You weigh advice from experts with regard to your own situation. You can simultaneously hold contradictory views and reason your way through to the direction you want to take. You have a personal agency that empowers your self-advocacy voice.

Susan's story gives an insightful glimpse into the complex health situation of what to do about the debatable issue of hormone therapy.

> *Although postmenopausal, Susan was still experiencing menopausal symptoms at age 54. Three months after I saw Susan for symptoms of hot flashes and night sweats, she was still feeling miserable despite black cohosh, acupuncture, and a clean diet without alcohol. The hot flashes and night sweats were disrupting her work and had become intolerable. Thinking she needed hormone therapy, Susan sent me an online message through the patient portal, asking for a prescription.*

While feeling sympathetic about Susan's misery and desire to feel better imme-diately, Carolyn informed Susan that the risks and benefits of hormone therapy needed to be discussed in greater depth than online messaging allows. Susan agreed to an in-person appointment but repeated that she was desperate and hoping for a quick fix.

> During our appointment, Susan seemed in a quandary, expressing conflicting beliefs and feelings. "I know I need hormone therapy, but I was hoping to do this naturally. But I have tried everything, and nothing is helping." Susan's fears had also been reinforced by a friend's opinion: "Oh, you don't want to take hormones—they can cause breast cancer. Medications are not natural." When I asked Susan to share her concerns about taking hormones, her list was typical of what I have heard from many women:
>
> - I feel like a failure if I "give in" to medication. Menopause is a natural process that I should be able to control. I am disappointed in myself for not being able to manage these symptoms.
> - I am not the kind of person who takes medication. Both my mother and sister went through menopause without hormones.
> - I'm worried about the risk of breast cancer, even though nobody in my family has had breast cancer, and the Women's Health Initiative study reassured me that the increased risk of breast cancer in the first few years is low.

Susan typically did not make rash decisions about her health. However, in this situation, her emotional and physical stressors were calling to her survival brain for help. She had to advocate for herself, right now and forcefully. Susan felt conflicting emotional tugs in shifting from a person who does not need medication under any circumstance to a person who uses medication to improve her life. Making the shift was difficult because her *subjective knower* part was listening to messages (heard and perceived) from her friend, mother, and sister.

Susan knew what she wanted to do to meet this challenge, but she could not do it alone. She needed Carolyn's medical support in reasoning her way through what, for Susan, was a complex situation fraught with emotions. Carolyn acknowledged Susan's conflicting feelings, asked questions, and listened carefully to Susan's responses to help her sort it all out. Susan was then able to make a decision. She accepted Carolyn's suggestion of a 3-month trial of hormone therapy to see if her symptoms would improve, while knowing that she could change her mind at any time.

Another patient, Polly, demonstrates constructed knowing in a long, winding journey after hip surgery went awry.

> Polly, age 75, had led an active life of hiking and camping until she fell and broke her hip. Nine months after hip replacement surgery, she was able to walk but with a significant limp and limited hip mobility. Frustrated that she could not resume her active lifestyle, Polly wanted to discuss her recovery with her surgeon. Unfortunately, because of the coronavirus pandemic, she had to wait several months for an in-clinic appointment. But she used her time well to prepare for her visit. She carefully made a list of direct questions to ask her surgeon about what could be done to increase her mobility. She also planned to request a referral for a second opinion about additional options for a fuller recovery. She even did her research on who she wanted to see for a second opinion and made sure her insurance would cover the consult. Polly's surgeon agreed that obtaining another opinion was reasonable and gave her a referral.

As these short examples suggest, the perspectives that can especially strengthen your advocacy voice are typically procedural and constructed knowing.

SUPPORTIVE SELF-ADVOCACY

Health issues are often scary and make us feel vulnerable. Going to a medical office can be overwhelming, especially if you are not feeling well. Having a trusted person with you can help you feel supported, communicate your needs, and help remind you later what the physician discussed and what directions he or she suggested. Be prepared with questions and concerns so these issues are addressed during your visit. Ask your friend to take notes or record the visit so that details can be revisited later.

Even women with the strongest self-advocacy voice know they are not meant to face these issues alone—and making sure you do not is an important part of self-advocacy. Ask for help and support, especially from family members and friends. Your relationships will also likely be strengthened by doing so.

Be aware that your ways of knowing come from multiple sources: how you feel (emotion), how you perceive (intuition), how you think (cognition), and how you act (conation). Your self-advocacy voice will be more powerful when you integrate these sources to support your body, mind, and spirit.

We want you to be well prepared to be a partner with your health practitioners. Rather than thinking of your physician or healthcare provider as the director of your health care, we encourage you to create your own network of practitioners who will make up your integrative-holistic team. This network is your personal *wellness web*. You are the center of that web, able to call on conventional and alternative practitioners when needed. Your wellness web should be dynamic, diverse, and evolving as your health improves and your horizons for healing expand.

3 Your Web of Wellness

We have presented women's ways of knowing as a framework for appreciating how and under what circumstances you should assert your advocacy voice. Unless you are fortunate to be part of a progressive integrative healthcare system, you will need to be both composer and conductor of the conventional and alternative practitioners in what we call your *web of wellness.*

Remember that in an integrative approach to care, you and your practitioners are partners in the healing process. However, you may have grown up during a time when the patient-doctor relationship was not seen as a partnership. Perhaps you know women who, regardless of accomplishment and competence in other aspects of their lives, view their healthcare practitioner as "the authority" and assume an uncharacteristically passive and vulnerable posture. Carolyn often hears patients say, "My blood pressure is normal at home but is always high when I come in to see you. I get so nervous coming to the doctor's office." We have all experienced the stress and anxiety of the medical environment. Carolyn has experienced it from both sides—as a physician and as a patient—and even she admits that she feels her heart racing and blood pressure rising while she sits in the exam room waiting for her physician, someone she has known personally and professionally for years.

RELATIONSHIP MODELS OF CARE

No doubt you are familiar with the traditional model, starring the doctor as authority. In this paternalistic relationship, the doctor tells you only what you need to know and what is best for you. An extreme example is Doc Martin from the PBS television series, who barks out orders and delivers news with absolute authority. Regardless of the manner in which instructions are delivered, this one-way relationship puts you in the position of *received knower.* There is no impetus, or maybe not even an opportunity, for you to engage in the process or advocate for what you want.

In today's society, patients have come to be thought of as healthcare consumers. In this approach, the physician-patient relationship is informative: you are provided facts and stats and then asked to decide what you want to do. For example, in the 30-minute follow-up appointment after a breast biopsy that revealed stage 1 cancer, a woman is told about treatment, including courses of chemotherapy, radiation, and medication. She is asked to consider joining a clinical trial and she is told about the oncotype test. Minutes before the end of the appointment, she is asked, "What do you plan to do?" Ready or not, this approach calls for *procedural knowing.* You are expected to use sharp reasoning skills to consider choices and make life changing decisions in a matter of minutes. It may be difficult for you to think clearly or rationally. It might be tempting to take an easier route, either going with your gut feeling or making the same decision that a friend has made in a similar situation. Although these tactics are not necessarily "bad," they are not likely to result in the most appropriate decision.

DOI: 10.1201/9781003250968-4

Relationship	Model of Care
Paternalistic	Authority
Informative	Consumer
Interpretive	Shared decision-making
Advocacy	Shared decision-making

An integrative-holistic perspective favors shared decision-making in the form of an *interpretive relationship*.[1] This approach calls on your *connected knowing* capacity. You are engaged in the process of receiving information and participating in making decisions. The practitioner's role is to translate information and data in ways that help you sort through options and make choices.

Although the interpretive relationship is a key part of shared decision-making, another aspect needs to be highlighted—that of your voice of self-advocacy. You, the patient, may want different kinds of emotional support or more in-depth deliberation about the pros and cons of treatment options. Or you may know exactly what you need and can guide your practitioner in your choices for how you would like your care to be managed. This is called an *advocacy-centered relationship*. You are the expert on your own life. As a constructed knower, you bring to the table awareness of your unique ways of knowing, emotional states, and life circumstances. In an advocacy-centered relationship, your practitioners will be curious about how you process information and arrive at decisions. They will be mindful that the conversation needs to be about more than just your physical health condition.

Here are the stories of three postmenopausal women in Carolyn's practice that illustrate two main points: the different tenors of how women express their advocacy voice, and the different ways that their voice is heard in the shared decision-making process. As you read these stories, consider what gets your attention and might speak to your own experience.

Maddy's story illustrates that self-advocacy can be a natural part of the process.

I had been seeing Maddy, age 72, as her primary care physician for many years. Maddy had a colonoscopy for severe digestive health symptoms that included persistent gas and bloating after eating. The results looked good, and the gastroenterologist told Maddy that nothing was wrong and not to worry. But Maddy's symptoms persisted, and she came to me for help. After we discussed Maddy's symptoms, I suggested that she see a functional medicine practitioner. Although Maddy was not familiar with this kind of practitioner, she trusted my judgment and was willing to explore a new route. She met with a practitioner her friend vouched for and felt confident in the recommendations, which included dietary changes, probiotics, and digestive enzymes. As her symptoms improved, Maddy was delighted to have found helpful options outside of conventional care as she expanded her web of wellness.

All too common among postmenopausal women is the diagnosis of breast cancer. These next stories are about two women with the same diagnosis who, in different ways, self-advocated and engaged in shared decision-making with their physicians.

Ana, age 55, and Becca, age 65, received the same diagnosis of stage 1 breast cancer. They were both advised that the standard of care is lumpectomy.

Ana consulted me, as her primary care physician, about her surgeon's advice to have a lumpectomy rather than the more aggressive route of mastectomy. However, Ana was quite clear that she wanted both breasts removed. She felt her mother might have lived had she chosen a mastectomy. Ana's reasoning: "I can accept not having breasts and do not need breast reconstruction at this time in my life." I gave Ana the name of a breast cancer survivor who had a bilateral mastectomy without reconstruction so she could have a private discussion with her and even see what post-surgery results look like. I suggested this might be helpful information before making her final decision. Ana followed through on my recommendation and then proceeded to have a bilateral mastectomy.

After learning about her treatment options, Becca declined all surgical intervention. She shared, "I've read that surgery can spread cancer. I do not want a lumpectomy. Keeping my body whole is central to my healthcare beliefs and removing that part of my body is not an option." In further discussion, I informed Becca there is no evidence that surgery spreads cancer. Nonetheless, Becca and her husband decided that a course of supplements, energy healing, and nutrition were in her best interest. We discussed the need for close surveillance and agreed on a follow-up appointment in 3 months for imaging and to revisit treatment options.

The stories of Maddy, Ana, and Becca reflect the need for and value of reflective dialogue between patient and physician. They underscore the tenets of integrative medicine: *attend to the person as a unique individual and understand her way of knowing.* This means that your practitioner sees you as a whole person and your physical condition in the context of your beliefs, emotional state, and life circumstances.

IMMUNITY TO CHANGE

Whether you are already an active participant in your integrative care or just starting to explore possibilities, being a partner in your own healthcare is likely to require some degree of change. To help you prepare for the second part of this book, which explains holistic options, it'll be helpful for you to think through where you are with regard to exploring and acting on alternative, integrative approaches as part of your health repertoire. Along with this, consider how prepared you are to engage in an advocacy-centered relationship with your providers.

We like the "immunity to change" model[2] because it raises the question of whether there might be a gap between your genuine intention to change something that is important to you and not being able to actually do it or to stick with it. In a general sense, immunity means keeping you safe—the purpose of your natural immune system is to protect you. Intentions that are positive and congruent with your beliefs enable you to move toward something and be ready to make changes. However, at times you might try to protect yourself from something that doesn't need protecting; you might actually be moving away from what you really want.

In the case of Hannah, treatment for stage 1 breast cancer included a lumpectomy, radiation, and an aromatase inhibitor. She wants to include working with a naturopath as part of her healing team. Let's follow Hannah's voice through the "immunity to change" four-step process:

- Stating intention
- Identifying limiting beliefs
- Examining protective beliefs
- Committing to action

NATUROPATHY

Naturopathy is a school of medical philosophy and practice that seeks to improve health and treat disease chiefly by assisting the body's innate capacity to recover from illness and injury. Naturopathic medicine is a "whole-systems" form of medicine that emphasizes prevention and individualized treatment of disease with lifestyle changes and natural therapies.

Step 1: Hannah states her intention as, *"I want to build up my immune system to enhance my healing process and remain healthy well into the future."* Note that Hannah states her intention in the affirmative. She is moving toward health rather than away from disease.

Step 2: Hannah has several limiting beliefs. She says, *"I believe there are big risks in going outside of conventional medicine, and the following concerns can keep me from focusing on my goal. I'm worried that my oncologist won't agree with me and might even abandon me. What if my conventional practitioners won't recognize the naturopath as a legitimate member of my care team? With the education and credentialing of naturopaths varying from state to state, what if the alternative practitioner I choose is not properly trained? Naturopath treatments are not as evidence-based as conventional treatments. Finally, I'm concerned that I will need to pay out of pocket because insurance doesn't cover naturopathy."*

Becoming aware of these concerns is an important part of the process. Now it's time for Hannah to probe more into her "hidden commitments," the more ingrained beliefs that also might inhibit her from making a desired change.

Step 3: Hannah examines her protective beliefs, considering what she is trying to protect. *"I want to protect my relationship with my oncologist, whom I do not want to alienate. I think about my reputation—I do not want to be ridiculed or thought of as the fool who goes to a nontraditional 'woo-woo' provider. Exploring an alternative path might also stir up the memories of the pain and trauma of my mother's death from breast cancer. I'm also concerned about my financial situation, feeling that I'm being selfish to invest dollars that my family could use elsewhere."*

Step 4: Hannah commits to action. She asks herself why and how much her intention to include naturopathy in her care matters to her. She thinks, *"I want to do the right thing for myself. I believe very strongly in listening to my body, and my intuition says to trust my body's innate ability to heal. The energetic and natural healing approach of naturopathy appeals to me. I want to exercise my voice, respect my intuition, and commit fully to self-care."*

Through working the steps of the "immunity to care" process, Hannah aligned her beliefs and intentions so she could take informed action. She decides to work with a naturopath and informs her other practitioners that the naturopath is a member of her care team.

You know from experience that while making significant changes is not an easy process, you have done it in the past and you can do it again. Just be aware that sometimes you are captive to your own immunity; when your brain is confronted with emotion-laden issues, it will do its very best to protect you. You can reach your goal when you open up your immune system—your beliefs—to energize the desired change. The most important element is to know why you set the intention in the first place and in what ways it is important to you. It's about you making the change you want for yourself.

How can you shift your immunity mindset toward beliefs and behaviors that will work in your best interest? Start anywhere and take the approach of incremental stacking. Concentrate on one modest change until it becomes a new habit. Add another and another until you are satisfied with the robustness of a particular pillar.

WELLNESS WEB

Holistic care seldom resides in one provider, one modality, or one discipline. Given the wide range of health conditions among postmenopausal women and your individual uniqueness, no single playbook will work for everyone. The opportunity is for you to create your own web of wellness that is customized to your particular and changing needs and to assert your voice of self-advocacy.

Think of your web of wellness as a network of providers, modalities, disciplines, strategies, and connections that support your health and keep you balanced. The web is likely to consist of both stable and fluid elements, depending on the state of your health at given points in time. It might help to picture a set of concentric circles. The inner circle represents the health providers who are your constants over a prolonged period of time. The middle circle includes those practitioners who are providing current and relatively recent modalities of care. The outer circle consists of providers who come and go, depending on your needs. We encourage you to include your own practices that nurture your body, mind, and spirit.

Your web may be simple or complex, linear, or multidimensional. It will look different for each woman depending on age, health status, and desire to create a comprehensive, integrative health network. The challenge is to take responsibility for developing and navigating a network of connections that will contribute fully to your health and well-being. It is helpful to first identify what is important to you as you age, and then educate yourself about the healing practices that exist within and outside of conventional medicine.

Part II

Expand Your Options

We believe strongly in whole-body health and integrated approaches to healing and wellness. In Chapters 4 through 11, we look at eight health conditions common in postmenopausal women that are amenable to integrative approaches: menopause, sexual health, sleep, anxiety, fatigue, weight, bone health, and brain health.

Because each woman's experiences of the realities of aging and health are unique, we offer an array of holistic pathways that you can pursue outside of, or in conjunction with, conventional medicine. We call this "bridging the gap."

As you read these chapters, be courageous and open-minded about some of the holistic approaches that you will encounter. Set your intention for an advocacy-centered relationship with your providers. Imagine creating a web of wellness that expands your repertoire of healing possibilities.

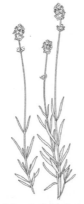

Lavandula angustifolia (Lavender)

DOI: 10.1201/9781003250968-5

4 Postmenopause
Restore Balance

Let's begin with Carolyn's own story (co-author). Her transition through menopause and beyond hit hard at an early age and, admittedly, was a big challenge. It started when she was 41, after a miscarriage.

> *I had hoped for a second child. Getting pregnant the first time had taken 2 years, so when I was pregnant the second time, I was overjoyed. When an early ultrasound showed no fetal heartbeat at 9 weeks, I was very saddened and disappointed but not surprised. I understood the risks of pregnancy at an older age. But I was surprised that after the miscarriage, my periods suddenly stopped. Then, within a few months, I began having hot flashes and night sweats. I realized that I was starting an early transition to menopause. The hot flashes were shockingly intense and extremely disruptive to my day-to-day activities, especially my work. I would be talking to a patient and suddenly—whoosh!—I'd flush with an overwhelming sensation of heat, beads of sweat erupting on my forehead, neck, arms, and abdomen. The episodes were so disquieting that concentrating on my work was difficult at times. I experienced an overall disruption of body and mind.*
>
> *As you are likely aware, a hot flash is more than just feeling warm or hot. The sensation of burning up from the inside out makes many women want to scream and rip off their clothes. But instead, somehow, we need to sit quietly and manage the overwhelming heat, sweat, and emotional dysregulation. While women describe the sensation in different ways, a common theme is a strong urge to flee one's own body. This experience was an awakening as I was forced to face the changes taking place in my body. I was soon to be on the other side of menopause at age 42!*
>
> *I have now lived 30 years as a postmenopausal woman and find life to be productive and purposeful . . . and I still have hot flashes.*

THE MENOPAUSE TRANSITION

Most of us will live a good portion—about one-third—of our lives beyond menopause. Every day about 6,000 women in the United States reach menopause age, and women reaching age 65 can expect to live, on average, for 20 more years. Being well informed about the life changes in these years after menopause will allow you to take charge of shaping how your future health will evolve.

Many women fear menopause because it means the loss of fertility. Cultural stereotypes about postmenopause reinforce a diminution of femininity and value. Just because you are no longer reproductive does not mean you are no longer productive. Far from being a tragic end to a vital life, the other side of menopause can be a gateway to new beginnings. It is a time to engage in self-care and to listen to your inner voice of knowing as well as the wisdom of women who have gone before. It is a time

DOI: 10.1201/9781003250968-6

to create an individualized approach to care that brings new understanding to your years after menopause.

WHAT TO EXPECT

Menopause is the time that marks the end of your menstrual cycles when you have gone 12 months without a period. Menopause can happen in your 40s or 50s, or more rarely in younger or older women. The average age of menopause for American women is 51. It is important to recognize that menopause is a natural biological process, just like going through puberty. It is not a disease but a transition to a new physiology, encompassing body, mind, and spirit.

Considering the type and severity of symptoms during the menopause transition, no wonder this time of life can be a major preoccupation. Resolution is neither predictable nor finite, and the length and intensity of symptoms vary from woman to woman.

Symptoms, such as hot flashes and night sweats, occur because of changing hormone levels that affect the body's temperature control. These vasomotor symptoms usually peak in the first 2 years after menopause but can last 5–7 years beyond your last menstrual period. Some women continue to experience vasomotor symptoms for 10–15 years or even lifelong.

Common Physical Changes and Symptoms Associated with the Menopause Transition

Irregular periods

Hot flashes

Night sweats

"Brain fog" (memory and cognition issues)

Insomnia

Mood disruption

Skin and hair changes

Many external factors are at play during menopause and beyond. You may be at the pinnacle of your career or launching a new one. Many women relate to the "sandwich generation," trying to balance the demands of caring for both children and aging parents. You may be experiencing relationship turmoil, career upheaval, unforeseen medical crises, financial stress—and the list goes on.

Do you remember the comic strip *Blondie?* Blondie's husband, Dagwood, was always making enormous sandwiches, filled with layers of meats, cheeses, and vegetables, all piled high and almost impossible to eat. We frequently see women attempting to eat the multilayered sandwich in one bite to get everything done. Not surprisingly, they become overwhelmed, immobilized, and discouraged. Frankly, it's impossible to get your mind around the whole. To be able to manage a "Dagwood sandwich," you need to cut it into small pieces. You may feel that taking care of everyone and everything else seems more important, but the essential ingredient in managing this transition through and beyond menopause is your own self-care. You must take time for yourself.

As you move through and beyond menopause, your body is taking on a new physiology, with a cascade of symptoms that can be subtle or overt. It is important to be aware of these changes so that you can communicate them to your healthcare practitioners and, in some cases, even educate your healthcare practitioners about the complexities of this life transition.

> *Martha, age 50, was an accomplished fundraiser for a nonprofit organization. In addition to dealing with the stress and anxiety of her pressure-filled job, she managed to raise two teenage daughters with a husband who was underemployed. She had always enjoyed good health, but during the last 6 months, she developed an intense burning sensation on the top of her head that would come and go and often trigger a debilitating headache. She sought advice from many physicians, had a brain MRI and tried various migraine medications. Nothing alleviated the pain or her other symptoms, which by now were interfering with both her work and home life.*
>
> *Martha came to me for an integrative medicine consult. While her symptoms were not the typical hot flashes and her periods were regular, given her age, her intermittent symptoms likely represented perimenopause. I thought that fluctuating hormone levels were triggering her symptoms and prescribed a low-dose estrogen patch. The burning on top of her head resolved within a couple of weeks, and Martha realized that her symptoms indeed indicated a perimenopausal state. Because she was concerned about breast cancer, she was not comfortable taking hormone therapy for any length of time. However, just knowing the cause of her symptoms was reassuring enough for her to go off the estrogen and commit to a daily mediation practice and regular exercise program to better manage the perimenopausal swings and anxiety. Martha commented appreciatively, "You made me feel like I was not crazy. So many previous physicians just minimized my symptoms and didn't consider fluctuating hormone levels as a cause."*

Feeling crazy and out of control is how many women describe this time of their lives. Please know that your symptoms and your feelings about them are both normal and unique to you. Being aware of how you are feeling is essential to finding ways to manage your emotional and physical symptoms. It will take time, attention, and sometimes medication.

PREGNANCY NO MORE!

Women often ask for confirmation that they have gone through menopause and are postmenopausal. However, this is not always easy to confirm from a clinical standpoint. The most important question is: *"When was your last menstrual period?"* The medical answer, which is often not very satisfactory, is: *"You are menopausal if you have gone more than one year without a period, with or without symptoms."*

What most women really want is proof that they are no longer fertile and cannot get pregnant. A blood test that measures levels of estrogen, as well as a reproductive hormone called follicle-stimulating hormone (FSH), may be helpful. A high FSH with a low estrogen level is highly suggestive of a postmenopausal state. Unfortunately, it is not always confirmatory, because these hormone levels can fluctuate greatly during the menopause transition. This means that results of blood tests can be confusing and not provide a clear answer. Nevertheless, blood tests can be valuable indicators of menopause status and prompt discussion and shared decision-making about your treatment options.

ESTROGENS AND PROGESTERONE

Estrogen is often thought of as a single hormone, but there are actually three notable forms: estrone (E1), estradiol (E2), and estriol (E3). E2, which is present in the body of women of reproductive age, declines to a very low level in postmenopausal women.

Estrogens	Natural Source
Estrone (E1)	Made by adipose fat, most prevalent in postmenopausal women
Estradiol (E2)	Made in the ovaries, declines dramatically after menopause
Estriol (E3)	Produced mostly during pregnancy

The declining levels of estrogen and progesterone contribute to the surge of symptoms associated with the menopausal transition. Hot flashes and brain fog are directly related to the fluctuating levels of estrogen. As estrogen and progesterone drop, hair grows more slowly and becomes much thinner. A decrease in these hormones also triggers an increase in the production of androgen. Androgens shrink hair follicles, resulting in hair loss on the head and, in some cases, can cause hair to grow on the face. This is why some women develop facial "peach fuzz" and small sprouts of hair on the chin. Loss of estrogen results in a decrease of collagen production, which affects changes in the skin. The fatty tissue between your skin and muscle lessens, so the skin loses its elasticity and is more fragile.

Long-term estrogen deficiency can also place women at higher risk of chronic conditions that can develop about a decade after menopause begins. For example, estrogen has a protective effect on heart health. When estrogen decreases, heart disease and high cholesterol can develop. Another example is the role of estrogen in the strength and density of bones. Estrogen helps in slowing bone loss, so the risk of osteoporosis increases when estrogen levels decrease after menopause.

Progesterone, a hormone that is naturally secreted by the ovaries, also declines as you transition through menopause. Lower levels of progesterone can contribute to headaches, mood disruption, and sleep issues. The loss of both progesterone and estrogen contribute to a hormone imbalance that is experienced during the menopause transition. Therefore, your body and brain need to rewire to establish a new equilibrium. Many strategies can help with this transition and the postmenopausal years that follow.

BRIDGING THE GAP

The transition to the other side of menopause is so individualized that you really do need to take charge of your own care. We recommend using an integrative approach to reclaim your equilibrium to help balance and manage your symptoms by listening to your body and assembling the right resources.

Although conventional healthcare practitioners certainly can be helpful during the menopausal transition, information and opinions vary greatly from practitioner to practitioner. Some may be willing to discuss hormones; others may not. Some may look outside the lens of conventional medicine and suggest alternative approaches; others may not. This is why you need to be equipped with an array of resources to address the issues that arise for you.

INTEGRATIVE STRATEGIES

HORMONE THERAPY

Let's talk about one of the most controversial and misunderstood treatments: hormone therapy (HT), or menopausal hormone therapy (MHT). Because hormone therapy can make a world of difference for some women in menopausal transition and beyond, it is an option to be considered. Hormone therapy was once seen as a common conventional approach to curb menopausal symptoms. However, many physicians are reluctant to prescribe it, largely because of research studies that dominated the news in the early 2000s (more on that later). But why aren't all women receiving up-to-date information about hormone therapy from their healthcare practitioners? The answer lies in a rather complicated story.

Regardless of where you are on the menopause continuum or your experience with hormone therapy, we think you'll find this backstory to be of interest, and you may want to share it with other women in your life.

The history of hormone therapy use goes back to the 1940s when Premarin, an estrogen replacement, was introduced to the market. Premarin is estrogen that has been isolated from horse urine, or conjugated equine estrogen (CEE). In fact, the name of the drug is short for PREgnant MARes' urINe.

Premarin became commonly prescribed because it was seen as a way to manage menopausal symptoms and significantly improve women's lives. Staying "forever feminine and youthful" was touted by some male physicians with sexist attitudes, who prescribed Premarin not only for symptom control but also to keep women youthful. By the 1970s, estrogen replacement therapy was firmly entrenched as the medical treatment for menopause; by 1975, Premarin was the most frequently prescribed drug in the United States.[1]

During this same time, the women's health movement was challenging medical authority by questioning the legitimacy of the disease model of menopause. The argument was that menopause was *not* a disease or sickness but a normal and natural process of aging. A landmark book, first published in 1971 by the Boston Women's Health Collective, *Our Bodies, Ourselves*, served as the most widely known health guide written specifically for women.[2] (The ninth and most current edition was published in 2011.) It offered more power and choice to women and signaled a new freedom of knowledge not dictated by male-dominated rhetoric.

Alternative opinions on menopause and hormone therapy started to circulate during the 1980s and 1990s. Michael Murray, ND, a naturopath, wrote *Menopause* to promote the natural approach to alleviate menopause symptoms.[3] Dr. Jonathan

Wright was one of the first physicians to write individualized prescriptions for hormone therapy using compounding pharmacies instead of FDA-approved, commercially available conjugated estrogens. In *Natural Hormone Replacement for Women Over 45*, Dr. Wright presented a template for how to prescribe compounded hormone therapy, which he suggested was safer than conjugated estrogens.[4] In another important book, *What Your Doctor May Not Tell You About Menopause*, Dr. John Lee advocated using a combination of natural estrogen and progesterone for hormone balance and disease prevention as opposed to using synthetic estrogen therapy.[5]

Until 2002, hormone therapy's wide usage was based primarily on observational data that suggested hormone therapy helped to prevent cardiovascular disease, support bone health, and relieve menopausal symptoms. It was the gold standard for relief of menopausal symptoms—that is, until the Women's Health Initiative (WHI) changed everything.

THE WOMEN'S HEALTH INITIATIVE

The WHI was launched in the late 1990s at 40 different U.S. sites. It was the first large, randomized, placebo-controlled trial designed to test whether hormone therapy, consisting of Premarin (CEE) and Provera (medroxyprogesterone), protected women from heart disease.

In August 2002, alarming preliminary results caused the WHI study to be stopped early because of an apparent increased risk of invasive breast cancer. News of this abrupt cancellation set off alarm bells in the medical community; consequently, many women were taken off hormones.

In June 2002, it was estimated that roughly 90 million prescriptions for hormone therapy were written annually. At that time, approximately 42% of women ages 50–74 were taking hormone therapy; that number decreased to 28% by July 2003.[6]

After the sudden halt to the WHI in 2002, both healthcare practitioners and women feared the use of hormones. Most physicians were no longer willing to prescribe hormone therapy, even if a woman was experiencing severe symptoms. However, as early as 2006, more in-depth analysis of the data indicated that a subset of younger women in the WHI did not show an increased risk of breast cancer. Findings from additional research demonstrated that hormone therapy started in the "window of safety" in the early menopausal years had relatively few risks and many benefits. For example, in women receiving estrogen and progestogen, breast cancer rates did not increase significantly until year 6, and in women receiving only estrogen, breast cancer rates were low and found to decrease.[7]

Unfortunately, during this period, medical education about hormone therapy was curtailed, resulting in practitioners being unprepared to manage hormone therapy in menopause. As recently as 2017, it was difficult for a menopausal or postmenopausal woman to find a physician willing to prescribe hormone therapy or even having sufficient knowledge to discuss menopause. In a 2017 survey of physicians in training,

---

Types of Hormone Therapy

HT   General overview abbreviation for hormone therapy

      Numerous FDA-approved hormone preparations are available for treatment of menopausal symptoms.

MHT   Current terminology is menopausal hormone therapy because it is more descriptive of its use.

      However, for the sake of simplicity, the term *hormone therapy* (HT) is used in this book.

ET   Estrogen therapy only

EPT   Estrogen and progesterone therapy

BHT   Bioidentical hormone therapy

      Preparations have exactly the same chemical and molecular structure as the estrogens and progesterone produced within the body.

34% indicated they would not offer hormone therapy to a symptomatic, newly menopausal woman, and a mere 7% reported feeling adequately prepared to manage their patients' experience of menopause.[8]

In the years since WHI, many women have been denied hormone therapy, including those with severe symptoms. Hopefully, this trend is changing as organizations like the North American Menopause Society (NAMS) continue their evidence-based training of health practitioners about risks and benefits of hormone therapy for the care of postmenopausal women. New and emerging information about safer approaches to hormone therapy are on the horizon as more research continues to unfold.

For the last 20 years, Carolyn's practice has been busy with women asking for integrated approaches for supporting good health after menopause, including appropriate prescribing of hormone therapy.

Lynn, age 56, made an appointment for a menopausal consult. She had her last period 2 years ago and hoped to avoid hormone therapy because her mother had breast cancer at age 65. Lynn was thin and active, exercised, ate well, and had a healthy relationship in a second marriage. Her two adult children were doing well on their own. She managed a healthcare clinic and frequently needed to give presentations to administrative and medical personnel. During these sessions, she would often experience a rush of heat in her face, and sweat poured down her forehead, neck, and chest. She could deal with the sweats, but "foggy thinking" made conducting a meeting challenging and often embarrassing.

Lynn was also irritable during the daytime because night sweats regularly interrupted her sleep. Her quality of life was poor. Her primary care physician had prescribed an antidepressant for her symptoms, but she did not think it helped much and it dampened her libido. When I heard Lynn's story, I suggested she consider hormone therapy to reduce her hot flashes and improve her quality of sleep. After discussing the risks and benefits—and the fact that her mother's breast cancer at age 65 did not put Lynn in a high-risk category—she agreed to give hormone therapy a try. She started on a low-dose transdermal patch of estradiol (E2), along with oral micronized progesterone. Within 2 weeks, Lynn was feeling well without hot flashes, and her sleep had markedly improved.

What is the difference between using a transdermal patch and taking estrogen in tablet form? In contrast to oral estrogen, the transdermal patches or gels deliver estradiol to the circulation at a continuous rate. Administering by the transdermal route avoids the drug being metabolized in the liver, which cuts down on the amount of drug available to the rest of the body and also decreases the risk of blood clots.

Bioidentical Hormones

The term *bioidentical hormones* originated in the alternative health vernacular and initially met significant resistance from the medical community. Admittedly, the term *bioidentical* can be confusing because it means different things to different people. Depending on the circumstances, it could mean natural, nonsynthetic, compounded, plant derived, or identical in chemical structure to the human hormone.

The actual definition of bioidentical means "compounds that have exactly the same chemical and molecular structure as hormones that are produced in the human body." Bioidentical hormones are plant based, primarily derived from soy and wild yam. To be therapeutic, they need to be converted to estrogen and progesterone in the lab. It is becoming more common for women's health practitioners to use bioidentical hormone therapy, reasoning that hormones should be replaced with a product that is closest to what a woman's body previously produced naturally.

Many FDA-approved bioidentical hormones are on the market. For example, estradiol (E2) is preferred by many practitioners as a first-choice bioidentical estrogen. The addition of progesterone to estrogen therapy is needed if a woman has a uterus to prevent uterine cancer. Progesterone in the form of micronized progesterone (Prometrium) is a commercially available, FDA-approved, bioidentical product. Progestins and progestogens are synthetic progesterone.

Bioidentical Products	Non-Bioidentical Products
Estradiol (E2), eg, Estrace	Conjugated equine estrogen (CEE), eg, Premarin
	Synthetic conjugated estrogen, eg, Cenestin
	Esterified estrogen, eg, Menest
Progesterone (micronized), eg, Prometrium	Progestins/progestogens
	Medroxyprogesterone acetate (MPA), eg, Provera

In France and other European countries, estradiol (E2) has been the estrogen of choice for hormone therapy, and it is becoming more widely used and studied in the United States. When prescribing hormone therapy, Carolyn typically starts with pharmaceutically manufactured, FDA-approved bioidentical products that contain estradiol (E2) and micronized progesterone. She does so because observational data suggest that this specific combination may confer a lower risk of breast cancer than that seen with the non-bioidentical combination (CEE + MPA) used in the WHI. However, further study is needed to confirm these findings.

Hormone Therapy Products Approved by the FDA

Product/Brand Names	Estrogen Type	Formulation/Administration*
Oral Estrogens		
Premarin	Conjugated equine estrogen (CEE)	Take 1 tablet daily (various dose strengths available).
Menest	Esterified estrogens	
Estrace	17-β-estradiol	
Transdermal Estrogen-Only Patches		
Alora, Climara, Menostar, Minivelle, Vivelle-Dot	Estradiol	Apply patch once or twice weekly to lower abdomen, upper buttock area, or outer hip (various dose strengths available).
Other Transdermal Estrogens		
Elestrin	Estradiol	Apply 1–2 pumpfuls of gel daily to upper arm and shoulder.
EstroGel	17-β-estradiol	Apply 1 pumpful of gel to inside and outside arm daily.
Divigel	Estradiol	Apply 1 packet applied daily to upper thigh.
Evamist	Estradiol	Apply 1–3 sprays daily to forearm.
Combination of Estrogen and Progestogen		
Premphase	CEE (continuous) plus MPA** (cyclic)	Take 1 tablet daily.

* Follow specific dosage instructions as provided by your practitioner.
** Medroxyprogesterone acetate
Modified, with permission, from Westberg SM. Menopausal symptom management. In Dixon DL, Harris IM, eds. *Ambulatory Care Self-Assessment Program*, 2021 Book 2. *Women's and Men's Care*. Lenexa, KS: American College of Clinical Pharmacy, 2021.

Compounding Pharmacies

Some women and practitioners mistakenly believe that bioidentical hormones are available only from a compounding pharmacy. The truth is that bioidentical hormones that are FDA approved (and typically covered by insurance) can easily be prescribed by licensed practitioners. Using a compounding pharmacy is an option when there is a need for a customized product with various bioidentical estrogens and progesterone in different amounts. These formulations contain pharmaceutical-grade, plant-derived estrogens, meaning that they are made to a high standard of purity; however, because they are individual, customized products, they are not FDA approved.

The use of products from compounding pharmacies can be helpful, particularly if you are allergic or sensitive to commercially available products or if a dose modification is not available in a standard FDA-approved product. As an example, estriol (E3)

Examples of Compounded Hormone Products

Preparation	Ingredients
Estrogen vaginal cream	Estriol (E3) or Estradiol (E2)
Bi-estrogen topical cream	Estriol (E3) + Estradiol (E2)
Bi-estrogen + progesterone cream	Estriol (E3) + Estradiol (E2) + micronized progesterone

---

vaginal cream is not available commercially, so it needs to be made in a compounding pharmacy. Also, for older women, insurance often does not cover FDA-approved estrogen vaginal cream so obtaining this product from a compounding pharmacy can be more affordable.

When Is Hormone Therapy Recommended?

In 2017, the North American Menopause Society (NAMS) published a Position Statement on the Use of Hormone Therapy.[9] NAMS based their position on an updated analysis of the WHI study that reported no increased risk of mortality in women who had been on different treatments: conjugated equine estrogen (CEE) with medroxyprogesterone acetate (MPA) over 5 years, or CEE alone over 7 years. The evidence illustrated that hormone therapy is the most effective treatment for hot flashes and vaginal dryness. NAMS recommends that for women younger than 60, or who are within 10 years of menopause onset, the benefit of treating bothersome hot flashes outweighs the risks for those without contraindications to hormone therapy. For women older than 60 who are initiating hormone therapy, or who are more than 10 years from menopause onset, the benefit-risk ratio is less favorable because of the increased risks of coronary heart disease, stroke, venous thromboembolism, and dementia.

Remember, there is no one size that fits all. Decisions about the type, dose, formulation, route of administration, and duration of use of hormone therapy should be based on your unique health risk, age, time of menopause, and goals of the therapy.

Risks and Benefits of Estrogen-Only Versus Combination (Estrogen-Progestogen) Therapy

The relationship between cardiovascular health and hormone therapy can change depending on the situation. The risk of coronary heart disease is possibly reduced if therapy is started at the time of menopause—the critical window of safety. However, if therapy is started 10 years or longer after menopause, the risks of heart disease, ischemic stroke, and blood clots are likely increased.

The situation is mixed for the outcomes on cancers that are common in women: breast, ovarian, and endometrial. With regard to breast cancer, the debate over the influence of hormone therapy remains somewhat unsettled. Consider the larger context that one in eight women will develop breast cancer during her lifetime. Hormone therapy adds very little risk of breast cancer, although the risk is likely to increase with longer use. For example, the WHI study found that the risk of breast cancer is decreased with estrogen-only therapy, while the risk is increased with combination therapy after 5 or more years of treatment. In the case of ovarian cancer, the risk may also increase slightly with extended duration (5–10+ years) of therapy with either estrogen-only or combination therapy. With regard to endometrial cancer, the risk was increased with estrogen-only but no different from baseline for combination therapy because progesterone protects the endometrium.

Before moving on, we pause to acknowledge that hormone therapy as treatment for menopausal symptoms remains controversial. Some doctors and other practitioners exercise caution by waiting for additional evidence-based research about the risks and benefits before they prescribe or recommend hormone therapy. Others, including Carolyn, base their recommendations, individual-by-individual, on available research evidence and on years of experience witnessing how hormone therapy can significantly help women manage symptoms and improve their quality of life.

We emphasize that hormone therapy is not for everyone and that every woman needs to be her own well-informed advocate. All potential risks and benefits must be weighed in a context of shared decision-making.

As an example, Maya sought advice regarding the risks and benefits of hormone therapy because of her menopausal symptoms.

Maya, age 52, was struggling with frequent hot flashes and night sweats and felt that her symptoms were exacerbating depression. She wanted to start on hormone therapy but was concerned because her mother had been diagnosed with breast cancer at age 56, and her older sister, at age 50. Both mother and sister tested negative for the BRCA gene. She had two other sisters without breast cancer.

Having two first-degree relatives with breast cancer, Maya was considered high risk. She was a candidate for high-risk breast cancer screening with mammograms alternating with MRIs every 6 months. So, what about hormone therapy?

I asked Maya, "If you started hormone therapy and, God forbid, one year later developed breast cancer, would you blame the hormone therapy?" She replied, "Of course I would, and I would never forgive myself for taking the estrogen." Given Maya's response, hormone therapy seemed out of the question. Instead, I advised other strategies for minimizing hot flashes and recommended other treatments for her depression.

If Maya had raised other concerns, the situation might be different. She might have said, "Dr. Torkelson, my quality of life is poor. I'm miserable, and I want to try a low dose of estradiol and see how I feel. Plus, I will continue with my high-risk breast cancer screening every six months." In that case, I would have recommended a trial of hormone therapy as a way to control Maya's symptoms.

When Carolyn is unsure if hormone therapy will be beneficial because a woman is not experiencing the classic symptoms of hot flashes and night sweats, she often suggests a short trial of hormone therapy. Such an exercise can clarify whether or not a true relationship exists between symptoms and hormones.

Judy was struggling with fatigue and low energy since reaching menopause. She was diligent about her exercise program and had reduced her work schedule in hopes of improving her daytime fatigue. Her sleep study was normal, and she had no night sweats or hot flashes. After a 3-month trial of hormone therapy with no improvement or change in symptoms, Judy and I agreed to discontinue it. Judy was experiencing lots of vaginal dryness and associated painful intercourse, although she thought the hormone therapy had helped a bit with that. So I prescribed a low-dose estrogen cream to relieve her vaginal dryness and alleviate painful intercourse, thus avoiding the systemic effects of an oral estrogen or transdermal patch.

When fatigue and quality of life do not improve with hormone therapy, as in Judy's case, it is time to look at other influencers in body physiology that can play a role. It is important to consider the extensive role that the hypothalamus-pituitary-adrenal-thyroid (HPAT) axis plays in how the endocrine system influences the body. A state of chronic stress (fight and flight response) can trigger cortisol that causes an array of imbalance in the levels of neurotransmitters and hormones. Finding ways to calm mental and physical stress is essential to managing menopausal symptoms and life beyond.

HPA Axis

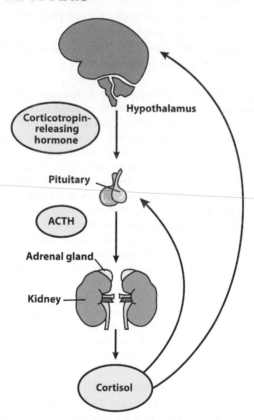

Reprinted with permission © 2020, Jones C, Gwenin C. Cortisol level dysregulation and its prevalence—Is it nature's alarm clock? *Physiological Reports* published by Wiley Periodicals LLC on behalf of the Physiological Society and the American Physiological Society.

This is when you might consult with a functional medicine practitioner, who will take an extensive history and order additional lab tests to look at underlying dysfunction in the HPAT axis. Testing the saliva and urine for cortisol, estrogens, and neurotransmitters can help get to the root cause. Once these results are known, the practitioner can recommend specific routines, foods, and/or supplements to correct the dysregulation and, in turn, maximize your health and comfort during this major life stage.

Duration of Hormone Therapy

Women who begin to have hot flashes early in the menopausal transition are at particularly high risk of having them occur for years. About 20% of women in their late 50s, 10% of women in their 60s, and 5% of women in their 70s experience persistent hot flashes. A minority of women remain highly symptomatic and require long-term, or even lifelong, hormone therapy to maintain quality of life. Shared decision-making, along with thinking of risks on a continuum (from low risk to high risk), can be helpful when considering hormone therapy.

> *Teresa, age 62, had been on hormone therapy for 14 years. On multiple occasions she had tried to wean off, but her hot flashes and night sweats would return within a couple of weeks. Determined to get off hormone therapy, Teresa stayed off for 2 months, but her symptoms did not diminish, and she begged to go back on. We reviewed the risks and benefits of hormone therapy and decided together that the best option for Teresa was to continue on the lowest dose of the estradiol patch to manage her symptoms and support her quality of life.*

A challenge for you and your practitioner is that once you are over age 65, it is much more difficult to get insurance to cover estrogen therapy. The low-dose estrogen patch, while ideal, is especially difficult to get covered, so looking at other less expensive options may be necessary. Using a compounding pharmacy can be a good alternative. Although compounding pharmacies do not make estrogen formulations in a patch form, a topical estrogen (E2 and E3) can work well. Finding the right dose for symptom control often is a trial-and-error process. Some integrative practitioners follow blood, saliva, or urine testing to determine the dosage of hormone supplementation.

Your practitioners should have up-to-date, evidence-based knowledge of hormone therapy. You may want to guide them to the North American Menopause Society, which is on the forefront of validated information. The 2017 Position Statement on the Use of Hormone Therapy provides a comprehensive review of the WHI and is updated as new research becomes available. As you consult with your practitioners, keep in mind that hormone therapy should be used at the lowest possible dose necessary to manage symptoms for the shortest amount of time. You should plan on making an annual visit to discuss risks and benefits to adjust the length of your hormone therapy as needed.

**NAMS RECOMMENDATIONS ON LENGTH
OF HORMONE THERAPY**

- For women 60 or older or who are within 10 years of menopause onset and have no contraindications, the benefit-risk ratio is most favorable for treatment of bothersome vasomotor symptoms and for those at increased risk of bone loss or fracture.
- For women who initiate HT more than 10 or 20 years from menopause onset or are 60 or older, the benefit-risk ratio appears less favorable because of the greater absolute risks of coronary heart disease, stroke, venous thromboembolism, and dementia.
- Longer durations of therapy should be for documented indications such as persistent vasomotor symptoms or bone loss, with shared decision-making and periodic reevaluation.

Not all women can or want to take hormone therapy to alleviate symptoms that impair quality of life such as brain fog and persistent hot flashes. If this applies to you, don't despair. Current research is investigating novel agents such as development of nonhormonal drugs designed to interrupt a specific chemical pathway thought to be involved in hot flashes. And you need not wait on the sidelines for new drugs to appear on pharmaceutical shelves. We suggest other ways to reclaim your equilibrium and feel better as you move through menopause and beyond.

FOOD, SUPPLEMENTS, AND BOTANICALS

Food, supplements, and botanicals are options to consider when looking to enhance your health. First, let's talk about foods. Diet and anti-inflammatory foods are not often brought up for discussion by gynecologists or primary care physicians during a routine visit. Yet, observations of menopausal experiences of women around the world suggest a link between menopause symptoms and diet. Menopausal symptoms differ in different cultures. Hot flashes, for example, have been reported by only about 10% of women in China, 18% in Singapore, and 22% in Japan. These statistics are in sharp contrast to those in Western cultures, particularly the United States, where hot flashes are experienced by 75% of women older than 50.[10] Research suggests that the Asian diet, which is primarily plant based, rich in rice and soy, and low in animal fat, may contribute to fewer menopausal problems than in Western countries, where an animal-based diet is common.

Whatever the specific reasons, it does seem that diet can have an impact on menopausal symptoms as well as on your general health after menopause. Certain foods are foundational, meaning they are important to incorporate into your daily meal planning. In contrast, you should avoid foods that may exacerbate or trigger symptoms.

Take note if certain foods bring on symptoms like hot flashes, night sweats, mood swings, or urinary frequency. Common culprits include sugar-filled or spicy foods, alcohol, and caffeine. Do you find that after a breakfast of a donut and coffee, or a glass of red wine in the evening, your hot flashes and night sweats flare? If so, once you know this is the case, you can take action by avoiding these triggers. We empathize—even when you know that certain foods and drink can make symptoms worse, habits are difficult to change. That voice of "immunity to change" (discussed in Chapter 3) might interfere with making shifts that will not only dampen the symptoms of menopause but also support and benefit your overall health.

Antioxidants and Cruciferous Vegetables

As you consider foods that are beneficial, we advise you to follow the age-old adage to "eat your veggies." Vegetables have antioxidant value and are low in calories, which helps manage weight and support healthy physical and mental well-being. Cruciferous vegetables are essential because they are rich in vitamins (folate and vitamin K), minerals (selenium and calcium), phytochemicals (plant sterols and indole-3-carbinol), and essential sulfur-containing compounds (called glucosinolates). The health benefits of cruciferous vegetables have been studied extensively. Many of the compounds in these vegetables synergistically contribute to health promotion such as anti-cancer, anti-inflammatory, and antioxidant capacities. Some studies have suggested that indole-3-carbinol (active metabolites in cruciferous vegetables) strongly influences estradiol metabolism and may be a new approach to prevent estrogen-dependent diseases. If you can make just one change to your diet, start by adding one serving of cruciferous vegetables to your daily meal plan.

Antioxidants are substances that may protect your cells against free radicals. These are natural by-products of metabolic processes, but when they build up, they can be harmful to body cells and results in oxidative stress (an imbalance between free radicals and antioxidants). By eating more plant-based foods, you supply your body with antioxidants that can help neutralize free radicals and reduce the risk of chronic diseases.

Cruciferous Vegetables

Arugula	Cauliflower
Bok choy	Collards
Broccoli	Kale
Brussel sprouts	Radishes
Cabbage	Watercress

Foods High in Antioxidants

Artichokes	Grapes
Beans	Kale
Beets	Orange vegetables
Berries (strawberries, blueberries, goji berries, raspberries)	Pecans
	Red cabbage
Cherries	Spinach

What About Soy?

The soybean, a species of legume originally native to East Asia, has for millennia held an important place in Asian cooking and culture. Only in the last hundred years has the soybean entered Western diets.

Soy, in its natural form, can be an excellent food source of protein, fiber, and isoflavones, all of which provide health benefits. The isoflavone metabolites of soy mimic estrogens in the body. Whether they help reduce hot flashes remains disputed in research, but in clinical practice, soy has been helpful for some women.

In a study published by the North American Menopause Society in 2021, a plant-based diet rich in soy reduced moderate to severe hot flashes from nearly five per day to fewer than one per day.[11] During the 12-week study, nearly 60% of women became totally free of their moderate to severe hot flashes. The diet in the intervention group consisted of a low-fat, vegan diet that included half a cup of cooked soybeans daily.

Women often wonder about the safety of eating soy. There is no evidence that soy causes cancer or that women with breast cancer should avoid eating soy foods. This was news to Catherine, who, like so many other women, was told by her oncologist to "never have soy," not even in her latte coffee. This erroneous belief came out of studies in the 1990s that showed isoflavones increased the growth of cancer cells in mice that had been genetically modified to develop breast cancer. Over the past 10 years, extensive research has clarified that soy does not increase cancer risk in women.

So, yes, you can add moderate amounts (1–2 servings a day) of soy foods, such as tofu, soy milk, or edamame, to your diet. As an example, a good protein intake is about 1 gram of protein per kilogram per day. A woman who weighs 70 kg (or 154 pounds) needs approximately 70 grams of protein a day, of which soy can be a part (one serving of tofu has about 14 grams of protein). Isoflavone supplements, on the other hand, contain higher levels of isoflavones and are generally not needed. Rather, eat the whole food source if you are going to consume soy. Note that some people do have a soy intolerance, so be aware of how your body responds to soy products.

Why Eat Organic Food?

This is a good time to talk about the benefits of eating organic food. The main reason is to minimize your exposure to environmental toxins. Although the integrative and naturopathic community has recommended organically and locally grown food for the past few decades, conventional medicine has never done so. However, a recent study published in the *Journal of the American Medical Association* found that a

---

The "Dirty Dozen"

Apples	Nectarines
Bell peppers	Peaches
Celery	Pears
Cherries	Spinach
Grapes	Strawberries
Hot peppers	Tomatoes

---

higher frequency of organic food consumption was associated with a reduced risk of cancer.[12]

Certain foods are known to have the most pesticide residues—the "dirty dozen." So at the very minimum, for these foods, you should select organic and, if possible, shop at your local farmers market where you can get locally grown products from farmers that use good farming practices. Although these food items may not be officially certified organic, they are likely better than those stocked in your local big box grocery store.

Supplements

We encourage you to get as many of your vitamins and minerals as possible from whole "real" foods. However, if you suffer from certain chronic conditions or if your diet is not optimal, supplements are sometimes necessary. And for everyone, there are two supplements that are hard to get from diet alone, and we encourage you to take them on a regular basis.

Vitamin D: Our body produces vitamin D from direct sunlight to the skin. However, most women do not get adequate sun exposure, especially women living in the northern hemisphere, women who limit their sun exposure to reduce the risk of skin cancer, and/or women who cover their bodies for religious or other reasons. Other women who are at higher risk of not having enough vitamin D are those who are overweight/obese, presumably because this fat-soluble vitamin is not as available to the body, and those with darker-pigmented skin because they are less able to synthesize vitamin D in response to sunlight. Therefore, supplementation with vitamin D is essential.

Vitamin D is necessary for a multitude of benefits as we age because it affects more than 30 body tissues, including hair follicles, reproductive system, and immune cells. Low serum levels of vitamin D are correlated with several metabolic conditions, such as increased triglycerides, low HDL cholesterol, and high blood pressure.[13] Vitamin D is also critical for maintaining bone integrity after menopause because it regulates the balance between levels of calcium and phosphorus in the blood.

A recent study out of San Luca Hospital in Milan, Italy, found that vitamin D levels were lower in adults hospitalized with COVID-19 than in those who had a mild case.[14] Additionally, having a low vitamin D level was associated with higher odds of ICU admissions.

The official recommended dose of vitamin D for postmenopausal women is 800 IU per day. But many other healthcare providers, including Carolyn, recommend 1,000–2,000 IU per day. Why? In clinical practice, Carolyn observes low levels of vitamin D, which suggest that either women are not taking it daily or the vitamin is not being absorbed correctly.

The normal range of a vitamin D level is 20–80 ng/mL, so over 40 ng/mL is ideal for maximum health benefits. For example, if a woman takes 1,000–2,000 IU daily, her vitamin D level will be around 30–40 ng/mL. If she takes 5,000 IU daily, her level will be around 60–80. If for some reason, you find you can't take vitamin D every day, taking a higher dose (such as 5,000 IU) a couple of times a week may be a more convenient option. Unless advised by your practitioner, taking more than 5,000 IU daily is not recommended because this fat-soluble vitamin can be stored in fat cells with unclear risks to health.

Fatty Acids: Omega-6 and omega-3 are called essential fatty acids because they must be consumed in the diet given that the body does not produce them. Both these fatty acids are important components of cell membranes and are precursors to many other substances in the body such as those involved in regulating blood pressure and inflammatory responses.

A ratio of omega-6 to omega-3 fatty acids of 4:1 is ideal. But the typical Western diet has a ratio of about 15:1, with excessive amounts of omega-6 fatty acids and insufficient omega-3. Therefore, decreasing consumption of foods high in omega-6 fatty acids (vegetable oils, meat, and poultry) and increasing consumption of foods high in omega-3 fatty acids (fish, flaxseeds, walnuts, and green vegetables) can promote a much healthier ratio. Balancing the ratio of omega-6 to omega-3 fatty acids is important because it can reduce the risk of diabetes, heart disease, obesity, metabolic syndrome, high cholesterol/triglycerides, and high blood pressure.

The usual recommended dose of omega-3 fatty acids is 1–3 grams daily. Getting omega-3 in adequate amounts in the diet can be a challenge, so adding a daily supplement may be necessary. Ground flaxseed is a good source of omega 3-fatty acid and is a suitable alternative if you find it difficult to take a fish oil supplement. You can easily add ground flaxseed to your diet by adding about 2 tablespoons to a smoothie or sprinkling the same amount over cereal or salad.

If you are concerned that you are not getting enough fatty acids, specialty labs can test for your omega-6 to omega-3 ratio to determine if you need additional supplementation.

Foods High in Omega-3 Fatty Acids			
Food	Amount (mg) Per Serving	Food	Amount (mg) Per Serving
Anchovies	951	Mackerel	4,107
Caviar	1,086	Oysters	370
Chia seeds	5,060	Salmon	4,123
Cod liver oil	2,682	Sardines	2,205
Flax seeds	2,350	Soybeans	1,241
Herring	946	Walnuts	2,570

Minerals: Many minerals are vital for maintaining healthy aging and metabolic functioning. Zinc, for example, assists in many hormone activities and is critical to immune function. Supplementation at 15 mg a day is advised for postmenopausal women. Likewise, manganese helps with carbohydrate metabolism and bone development and is important in a wide range of metabolic functions, including its role as a cofactor for a number of enzymes important in energy production and antioxidant defense. The many food sources for manganese include mussels, wheat germ, tofu, sweet potatoes, nuts, brown rice, lima beans, chickpeas, spinach, and pineapples. Supplements typically provide 1 to 4.5 mg of manganese. Taking a complete mineral supplement daily is an easy way to ensure adequate intake.

Botanicals

Black cohosh is among the most thoroughly studied herbal medicines that are used to treat menopausal symptoms. It is a perennial herb, native to North America, and a member of the buttercup family. It has been used traditionally for a variety of problems in women, including pain during childbirth, uterine colic, and dysmenorrhea. Because it has anti-inflammatory properties, black cohosh can improve joint health.

Although scientific evidence is lacking to support the use of black cohosh for menopausal symptoms, naturopaths have used black cohosh in combination with other herbs for years with clinical success in decreasing hot flashes. The dose generally recommended is 40–80 mg twice a day of a standardized extract. This is a situation when you will need to decide if you want to reach outside the conventional healthcare system to consult with a naturopath about botanical medicine as an adjunct to your care.

Siberian rhubarb was introduced from Germany, where it has been used for more than 20 years for hot flashes and other vasomotor symptoms. The product, sold as Estrovera in the United States, contains a proprietary extract called "rhaponticin" or "extract ERr 731." The herb has been used as a food and as a medicinal plant for constipation, diarrhea, and other gastrointestinal problems.

Curcumin is the main active ingredient in turmeric, naturally found in the root of the turmeric plant, which is an herbaceous perennial of the ginger family. Curcumin has antioxidant and anti-inflammatory effects that provide multiple health benefits. It aids in the management of inflammatory conditions, metabolic syndrome, arthritis, pain, and degenerative eye conditions. It may help in the management of exercise-induced inflammation and muscle soreness. In addition, a relatively low dose of curcumin can promote gut health, in people who do not have diagnosed health conditions. These benefits are best achieved when curcumin is combined with agents such as piperine (the chemical found in black pepper), which increases its bioavailability.

The dose of curcumin used in research studies ranges from 80 mg to as high as 1 gram. Supplements typically have 500 mg of curcumin per tablet, and your practitioner may recommend one or two tablets daily. Women often wonder if cooking with turmeric, the spice, could yield the same health benefit as its constituent curcumin. Turmeric has been used in both culinary and medicinal worlds for thousands of years. Yes, use it in your cooking.

Boswellia is a gum resin extracted from a tree that is native to India and Arabia. It contains anti-inflammatory compounds known as boswellic acids, which act to prevent the formation of certain pro-inflammatory chemicals, such as leukotriene and prostaglandin. Given its anti-inflammatory benefits, boswellia is used to support healthy joints and other inflammatory conditions.

Both curcumin and boswellia may be useful for postmenopausal women who have joint inflammation, muscle pain, or other inflammatory conditions. Many dietary supplement formulations contain two herbs because evidence supports a greater, or synergistic, effect when the two are used in combination.

Are Supplements and Botanicals Safe?

Approximately 166 million Americans take dietary supplements, spending $30 billion annually.[15] You may question: Should I be taking supplements, too? Are they regulated? How do I know if they are safe?

Dietary supplements are regulated as a special category of food, rather than as drugs. The Food and Drug Administration (FDA) has the authority to regulate companies that manufacture, distribute, and sell dietary supplements—and to take enforcement action against unsafe and mislabeled products. However, unlike the situation with drugs, the FDA does not evaluate and approve dietary supplements before they are marketed. Rather, the manufacturing company is responsible for determining that their dietary supplements are safe and that any representations or claims made about them are substantiated by adequate evidence to show that such claims are not false or misleading. However, to ensure better safety of these products, in 2007, the FDA established regulations and the authority to enforce what are called current Good Manufacturing Practices (cGMPs) for companies that manufacture, package, or hold dietary supplements. These regulations focus on practices that ensure the identity, purity, quality, strength, and composition of dietary supplements.

A few things to remember. First, dietary supplements are considered "foods." That means the way they are marketed is in the hands of each manufacturer, not the FDA. Therefore, when looking for a dietary supplement, we advise you to find a product that follows cGMPs. Often, naturopaths and functional nutritionists will carry products in their offices to ensure that their patients are getting the highest-quality product.

Second, consuming "real food" as the main source of your vitamins and minerals is always the best approach. However, as we've discussed, dietary supplements can play important roles in achieving optimal health for menopausal women. Before starting any supplements, discuss the issue with a provider who is knowledgeable and experienced with supplements, and who knows you, your history, and any medication(s) you take. This approach will help ensure you select the supplement(s) that are most appropriate for you, in the appropriate doses, and that are of good quality.

And third, it is also important to understand that something that is "natural" can still have potential side effects, including interactions with medications or other supplements. If you experience any side effects, you should report them promptly to your practitioner.

HEALING SYSTEMS

We believe there will be times when you could benefit from systems of healing that are outside the purview of conventional medicine. Your body has natural mechanisms for repair and healing. Two systems of healing that may help you improve your quality of life are traditional Chinese medicine/acupuncture and yoga.

Traditional Chinese Medicine and Acupuncture

Traditional Chinese medicine (TCM) is one of the oldest systems of medicine, practiced far longer than conventional medicine. TCM is based on the belief that vital energy, called *qi*, flows through the body and performs multiple functions to maintain health. Acupuncture is a component of TCM in which needles are inserted at specific points to rebalance energy flow.

Carolyn often refers women to an acupuncturist if they are unable or reluctant to take hormone therapy for their symptoms, or if they want to start with acupuncture as the first treatment strategy. Fortunately, many people in the integrative community are TCM/acupuncturists. These skilled practitioners and healers can offer tremendous support to women at all stages of the menopausal transition. In Chinese medicine, menopause is called "a second spring," the emergence of a transformation.

Brenda, age 58, expressed that she had been feeling "not myself." Her symptoms included a little weight gain, lower energy, mood irritability, and inability to concentrate. She was stuck and didn't know where to turn. She wasn't ready to try antidepressants. Because Brenda had no vasomotor symptoms and was postmenopausal for 3 years, I didn't think hormone therapy would be helpful. She already was seeing a therapist and working on past childhood trauma. She had not tried acupuncture in the past, so I referred her to an acupuncturist who works primarily with women.

Brenda reported that the acupuncturist worked on "lots of stuck grief" during her first appointment. This way of describing a health condition may sound weird or unconventional for some, but the acupuncturist worked on opening Brenda's lower chakras until the grief energy was able to pass through unimpeded. Following a series of treatments guided by her skillful practitioner, Brenda was able to restore a balance to her body. Most astonishing to me was Brenda's sense of relief and new-felt freedom. In addition, she now felt ready to work more intensely with her therapist on her childhood trauma.

Research supports the benefits of acupuncture on menopause-related symptoms. A statistical meta-analysis conducted on the results of 12 scientific studies, involving 869 participants, indicated that acupuncture significantly reduced the frequency and severity of hot flashes.[16]

To become a qualified TCM practitioner in the United States, 3–4 years of full-time postgraduate study at an accredited educational institution are required. Most states require national board certification by the Certification Commission for Acupuncture and Oriental Medicine. Because of research supporting the benefits of acupuncture, the introduction of acupuncturists into the healthcare system is becoming more accepted. We strongly advocate incorporating acupuncture into the healthcare delivery system, including coverage by insurance.

Yoga

Yoga refers to the union of mind and body. Yoga has been studied specifically for relieving menopausal symptoms. Results of a recent meta-analysis of 13 studies involving 1,306 participants showed that yoga improved *all* menopausal symptoms when compared with no intervention.

Various forms of yoga practice serve to calm the mind, help with stress reduction, and improve mood and concentration. In addition, yoga helps to increase strength and flexibility, balance and coordination, reaction times, lung function, cardiovascular conditioning, and weight loss. Yoga is undisputed as an adjunct intervention for menopausal and postmenopausal women.

Yoga is steeped in thousands of years of history and tradition. As the practice evolves, new styles are developed, and teaching approaches modified. Now there are many different kinds of yoga practices, so look for a style or a teacher that appeals to you. Keep exploring until you find the best fit.

Two traditional practices you might have heard of are Iyengar and Ashtanga, which focus on breath (*pranayama*) and posture (*asana*). Iyengar yoga is based in hatha yoga in which the student is guided by the teacher to focus on the nuances of each *asana* until proper alignment is achieved. Props such as blankets, blocks, straps, and bolsters are used to help students stay in good alignment. Iyengar is not a flowing style of yoga. Rather, each posture is held for extended periods while the student adjusts her body and corrects alignment, which help to build strength and stamina.

Ashtanga is a form of Vinyasa yoga, which means the postures are connected through flowing movements. The practice is a set sequence of postures performed in the same order every time. Each movement is done on the breath, and each posture builds on positions that come before it. A traditional series of movements called the Sun Salutations are often used as warm-up sequences in Ashtanga and Vinyasa yoga practices.

The goal of all yoga is to find a place of peace and calm. The specific type, such as Iyengar or Ashtanga, is less important than finding the style that works best for you. Be patient because it may take a bit of searching and experimenting.

> *Angela, at age 52, had tried everything, both alternative and conventional, to relieve her severe hot flashes and night sweats. Estrogen therapy did not improve her symptoms; in fact, her migraine headaches flared (remember, not all hot flashes are estrogen-responsive), and progesterone therapy made her more depressed. Her son had died the previous year, and although she was seeing a grief therapist to deal with the trauma, as well as exercising and eating a better diet, Angela remained miserable. We turned to the possibility of a meditation/yoga practice. She tried out different classes before landing on kundalini yoga, a style that involves chanting, singing, breathing, and repetitive postures. Angela's hot flashes—and her sexual relationship with her husband—improved. While yoga did not resolve all of Angela's symptoms, she did feel she had more control of her life.*

We encourage you to look at a variety of yoga options and see what resonates with you. If you are like most of us, you'll want to find a practice that is not too challenging yet still stretches and calms the body. Try different classes available in your

TYPES OF YOGA

Hatha yoga is a general category that includes most yoga styles. It is an old system that includes the practice of asanas (yoga postures) and pranayama (breathing exercises). The movement in hatha yoga classes is often done slowly, requiring you to hold each pose for a few breaths.

Iyengar yoga is a form of hatha yoga that emphasizes detail, precision, and alignment in the performance of posture and breath control.

Ashtanga yoga follows a set sequence of asanas, or poses, that are practiced the same way each time, holding each pose for five breaths. There are three series of poses, each with different focuses, that can be physically challenging.

Vinyasa yoga coordinates movement with your breath and movements that flow from one pose to another. Many types of yoga can also be considered Vinyasa flows, such as ashtanga, power yoga, and prana. Vinyasa was adapted from ashtanga yoga in the 1980s.

Bikram yoga is a system of yoga that Bikram Choudhury synthesized from traditional hatha yoga techniques. It became popular in the early 1970s. Classes run for 90 minutes and consist of the same series of 26 postures, including two breathing exercises.

Hot yoga refers to yoga exercises performed under hot and humid conditions, typically leading to profuse sweating. The purpose of the heat in hot yoga varies depending on the practice or the individual.

Kundalini yoga is a school of yoga that is influenced by Shaktism and Tantra schools of Hinduism. It is equal parts spiritual and physical. This style is all about releasing the kundalini energy in your body said to be trapped, or coiled, in the lower spine. It derives its name through a focus on awakening kundalini energy through regular practice of mantra, tantra, yantra, yoga, or meditation.

Yin yoga is a slow-paced style of yoga with postures, or asanas, that are held for longer periods of time. Its focus is on the balance of the mind and the body.

Restorative yoga uses bolsters, blankets, and blocks into passive poses so the body can experience the benefits of a pose without having to exert any effort. It is meant to relax and calm the mind and body.

community, various videos, Zoom classes, or YouTube, and begin to move. Really, any form of yoga and stretching will have benefits.

———————

Your story as you move through menopause and beyond is an opportunity to engage in holistic practices that will support your body, mind, and spirit. Your experience will be unique to you and supported by the many women who have come before you. Living your life on the other side of menopause is an exciting time to find new pathways for optimizing your health. You have the ability and capacity to make this happen.

PATHWAYS TO RESTORE BALANCE

Self-Awareness: You may be transitioning through an early or later stage of postmenopause. What in this chapter speaks to you and why? What have you learned that you didn't know before?

Self-Compassion: In what ways are you caring for yourself in postmenopause? Give yourself credit for the actions you have taken. What needs more healing?

Self-Advocacy: Which of the healing modalities might you add to your repertoire? What therapies might you benefit from during this period of your life?

———————

CATHERINE'S PATHWAY

Having been through the throes of "have or have not" concerning hormone therapy, I want to share some of my experience.

*To begin, I assumed that I would **not** be one of those women who suffered through menopause. At age 45, and to my surprise, my perimenopausal symptoms were severe enough to leave me feeling fatigued, irritable, fuzzy headed, and, quite unlike me, experiencing feelings of hopelessness. I tried to cope with these miseries while working full-time and living with my daughter during her onset of puberty. Eventually, I had to admit that managing on my own simply was not working. Although I was aware that the women's health movement encouraged a natural transition without hormones, I was open to hormone therapy given its promise to relieve my debilitating symptoms. With encouragement from my primary care doctor and gynecologist, I embarked willingly on a 12-year stint with an estradiol and progesterone combination hormone therapy. For the sake of my overall well-being, I felt the benefits would far outweigh the risks.*

Then, at age 57, I was diagnosed with estrogen-positive, early-stage breast cancer, and I was forced to stop hormone therapy. I needed to make myriad choices, all of which were accompanied by uncertainties and dilemmas, including type of surgery, radiation with or without chemo, participation in a clinical trial, etc. Ironically, the post-cancer medication triggered the same menopausal symptoms that I had experienced before hormone therapy. I endured these symptoms for 7 more years; once off the medication, the symptoms, except for sleep disruption, disappeared. I don't belabor the question of whether estrogen therapy increased my risk of breast cancer or perhaps caused it. Having good quality of life during those years on hormone therapy was so important to me that I can't imagine having chosen a different scenario.

Since 2007, I have been working weekly with a highly skilled personal trainer who incorporates yoga breath work and poses into my routine. I am satisfied with maintaining improvement in my posture, balance, and overall strength. As a constant seeker of calm and peace, the yoga-related work, along with acupuncture, keep me relatively well balanced.

5 Sexual Health
Energize Flow

With the television and film industry's portrayal of older women in vibrant, lead roles—from *The Golden Girls* of the 1980s to the more recent series *Grace and Frankie*—it's out in the open that older women have sex. And yes, they use vibrators! This is a heartening picture for sure, but is it true-to-life for most postmenopausal women?

Sex As We Age
National surveys tell a different story concerning women's sexual activity and sexual health as we age. According to the 2018 National Poll on Healthy Aging, 40% of men and women between the ages 65–80 reported being sexually active, most of whom with a romantic partner. The same poll revealed notable gender gaps. For instance, women were less likely than men to be sexually active: 31% versus 51%, respectively. The biggest gender difference was that half of the men ages 65–80 years said they were extremely or very interested in sex compared with just 12% of women in the same age range.[1]

Women interviewed for a longitudinal study on *Vital Women in Their 70s* offered candid perspectives on what sexual intimacy meant to them. Of the women who had a male partner, most preferred gentle touch rather than intercourse. Whether partnered or not, many of the women chose masturbation for orgasmic satisfaction. Other researchers interviewed 16 straight and 16 lesbian married couples to better understand sexual changes in midlife. In both groups, sexual activity and desire diminished over time due to health, aging, and caregiving events. Nevertheless, the lesbians described a stronger sense of duty to keep sex alive.[2]

Normal postmenopausal physical changes can affect sexual interest and sexual activity. The decrease in estrogen creates a collection of symptoms affecting the external genitalia, urethra, bladder, and vagina. As estrogen levels fall, cervical secretions decrease in amount and the vaginal lining becomes thin. As a result, at least 50% of postmenopausal women suffer from GSM—genitourinary syndrome of menopause—with symptoms of vaginal dryness, recurrent urinary tract infections, and painful sexual intercourse (dyspareunia).

GENITOURINARY SYNDROME OF MENOPAUSE (GSM)

GSM is a relatively new term for the condition previously known as atrophic vaginitis, or urogenital atrophy. This hypoestrogenic state causes chronic, progressive, vulvovaginal, sexual, and lower urinary tract conditions characterized by a broad spectrum of signs and symptoms.

DOI: 10.1201/9781003250968-7

Why do we care about a woman's sexual health as she ages? Because sexual health is important for your physical and mental well-being. During sexual activity, endorphins (neurotransmitters that can bring about positive feelings) are released and can reduce stress and help with sleep. The intimacy associated with sexual activity can enliven long-term relationships. Women who continue to be sexually active after menopause are less likely to have significant vaginal atrophy or thinning of vaginal walls: a use-it-or-lose-it phenomenon.

In Carolyn's clinical practice, many women express complaints about their sexual health such as: "I have no libido. I rarely have an orgasm anymore. I've stopped having sex because intercourse is too painful. I'm self-conscious of my changing body. My partner is not interested. I do not have a partner." The clinical setting, with your health practitioner, is the opportune time to address your concerns. Yet, in a survey of American women ages 57 to 85, only 22% reported they had discussed sexual health with a physician since they had turned 50.[3] If you are among that 22%, great! If you are in the group whose physician or other provider does not initiate the conversation, it's time to step into your self-advocacy boots. We recommend you start the conversation with whomever you feel most comfortable—your primary provider, gynecologist, acupuncturist, or other practitioners. Test it out by simply asking, "I would like to bring up a few concerns about my sexual health. Are you open to discussing them with me?" If not, look for someone else. There are many solutions to help improve these problems; integrative health is a fertile place to start.

BRIDGING THE GAP

The truth is that sexual health is rarely on the minds of most health practitioners when seeing a woman who is 60, 70, or 80+ years old. Considering the benefits of sexual health on our lives, this is a sad state of affairs. Although recent articles encourage practitioners to address the topic of sexual health with their patients, the postmenopausal woman as a sexual being is still often neglected in the conversation.[4]

We say it again: this is a time to make use of your self-advocacy skills. Be bold and brave. Talk with your healthcare provider about symptoms or issues that are concerning you. Engage in conversation with your partner about questions you want to explore. Begin the dialogue so that sexual concerns can be resolved, and you can enjoy sexual activity for years. Your sexual health should not be a forgotten component of aging. It is as fundamental as the food you eat, the exercise you do, or the friends you enjoy.

INTEGRATIVE STRATEGIES

CONTRIBUTING FACTORS AND CONDITIONS

Let's return to the question—*Why don't more women enjoy an active sex life?* Many factors can influence sexual inactivity. We describe five conditions individually; many women experience more than one.

Hot flashes: Studies have shown that severe hot flashes can negatively affect your sexual activity. Hot flashes can occur at any time and often show up in full force during bedtime hours. The sensation of heat brought on by hot flashes can be so intense and unpleasant that the prospect of sexual intimacy seems too distasteful. Being red and sweaty is not the same as being hot and sexy! Women who used to enjoy sleeping close to their partner may find that their partner's body heat triggers hot flashes and leads to distancing. For some couples, differences over what's a comfortable bedroom temperature can lead to sleeping in separate rooms. Many women continue to experience hot flashes well beyond menopause.

Painful intercourse: It's hard to feel desire for or have fun with intercourse if it's a painful experience for you. The decline in estrogen levels after menopause can cause a decrease in vaginal lubrication, loss of vaginal elasticity, and thinning of vaginal tissue. This results in a range of symptoms from vaginal dryness and tightness to sharp, shearing pain during penetration. Some women feel intense soreness or burning in the vulva or vaginal area after sex, even if intercourse is not painful. Upward of 45% of postmenopausal women report that intercourse is painful.

> *Kristine's story is common. She came to me in desperation: "What do I do? My husband insists on intercourse, and it's so painful I can hardly stand it. When I told him it hurts, he just said, 'Well, just do it for me then.' " Unfortunately, many men do not understand how painful intercourse can be for women with the loss of estrogen. Yes, Kristine was already using a lot of vaginal lubrication, but intercourse was still painful. I prescribed vaginal estrogen cream nightly for 3 weeks, advising Kristine that once intercourse was no longer painful, she could reduce the dose to two or three times a week.*

If you experience chronic vaginal dryness, despite the use of moisturizers and lubrication, you will likely need to use a low dose of vaginal estrogen therapy long term to continue having vaginal intercourse. Vaginal dryness, unlike hot flashes, does not go away over time. You need to keep those estrogen receptors in the vagina happy with a regular dose of estrogen. Another important factor is the use-it-or-lose-it phenomenon: regular sex, either with a partner, through masturbation, or a combination of the two, definitely helps keep vaginal tissues more supple and moist.

Keep in mind that having a healthy vagina and vulva is important, even if you are not having intercourse. For example, if you engage in "outercourse" (particularly if vaginal penetration is too painful), having vulvar lubrication is helpful. A rarely discussed condition is called "vaginal awareness," which develops in women who have vaginal dryness that causes constant irritation and a feeling of the presence of the vagina—and not in a pleasurable way. The good news is that there are treatments for these conditions.

For many women with vaginal dryness that is mild to moderate, lubricants and moisturizers can effectively relieve pain during intercourse. These products are the natural place to start and are available over the counter. If you have more severe vaginal dryness and related pain, or if lubricants and moisturizers don't work well for you, then you may want to consider vaginal estrogen. These prescription products deliver estrogen directly to the vagina, with minimal absorption to the rest of the body. In addition to supporting vaginal tissue, estrogen also may help to enhance arousal and improve orgasms.

Lubricants

Type	Examples
Water-based	Astroglide, FemGlide, Just like Me, K-Y Jelly, PreSeed, Liquid Silk, Maximus, Sylk, others
Silicone-based	I-D Millennium, Pjur, Pink, Pure Pleasure, others
Hypoallergenic and chemical-free	Free Pink® Made with silicone, vitamin E, Aloe vera, and Glycerin-free; Just Like Me; Good Clean Love 95% organic materials, paraben, and glycerin-free
Natural option	Coconut oil (can be used on outside of vaginal area)
Moisturizers	Replens, Luvena, Fresh Start, K-Y Silk-E, Moist Again, K-Y Liquibeads, others

Low libido: Women of all ages might report lack of desire, but it is even more present in postmenopausal women. Having a low sex drive is a complicated story given that most menopausal women do not have stores of estrogen, progesterone, and testosterone, all of which are needed to support their sexual health. Testosterone—which women have in lower levels than men—is most closely associated with libido and declines as a woman ages.

However, aging may not be the whole story. Another factor is medication, frequently prescribed for anxiety and depression, that can significantly dampen your libido. Examples include SSRIs (selective serotonin reuptake inhibitors), such as citalopram and fluoxetine, and SNRIs (serotonin–norepinephrine reuptake inhibitors), such as venlafaxine and duloxetine.

Life stressors, anxiety, and fatigue also can interfere with desire. Certainly, a poor relationship with your partner can lead to a lack of interest in sex. These are all factors that need to be considered if libido is to be improved.

A small percentage of women actually have an enhanced libido as they transition through menopause. One theory is that the sex hormone globulin, which binds itself to both estrogen and testosterone, declines when estrogen declines. Now there is less globulin to bind to the testosterone, which becomes freed up, and more is available in the body.

In an episode of *The Moth Radio Hour* on Minnesota Public Radio, a woman told a fascinating story about how her libido exploded as she went through menopause. She went on a hunt for men to have different sexual experiences that were new and exciting. She was not necessarily looking for a relationship but rather to explore the intense sexual feelings that had awakened in her body. While some women may wish for this kind of awakening (not necessarily the man-hunt part), most postmenopausal women struggle with a low libido that adversely affects many aspects of a relationship.

Difficulty with orgasm: According to various studies, 75% of women don't reach orgasm solely from intercourse and require sex toys, lubricants, and hand or tongue stimulation. Another 10%–15% of women don't climax at all. Even before menopause, the female orgasm is a complicated matter. After menopause, orgasm can become more difficult. For postmenopausal women, the decline in hormone levels means a decrease in blood flow to the clitoris and vagina, which reduces nerve sensitivity and can make orgasm more challenging to experience.

> *During a visit, a 65-year-old woman admitted she had never had an orgasm and said, "I want to have an orgasm before I die." Recently, she had been able to discuss this issue with her second husband after 20 years of marriage. With my encouragement, they sought the help of a sexual counselor to confront the problem head-on and resolve it.*

The good news is that women are blessed with bodies that are capable of experiencing orgasm in more ways than one. The most common type of orgasm is clitoral. Many women also experience orgasm through vaginal stimulation. Some women can have orgasms through stimulation of the breasts or other parts of the body, or through the use of sexual imagery without any touch at all. Researchers have even found a nerve pathway outside the spinal cord, through the sensory vagus nerve, that will lead a woman to experience orgasm through sensations transmitted directly to the brain. Many nerve pathways are responsible for the experience of orgasm in women. So be assured that sexual pleasure can be experienced in a variety of ways.

> *During her reproductive years, Norma's sexual activity had been limited to solo masturbation. At age 59, Norma began having intercourse with a male partner she met through internet dating. Soon he suggested that they have anal intercourse, which was not something Norma had ever imagined doing. During our visit, Norma was eager to raise questions and concerns about whether anal intercourse was appropriate and safe. At first, I was caught off-guard, but quickly realized that I needed to approach her questions with responsible and respectful answers. I said that while coital intercourse is the most common sexual behavior, anal intercourse also is an expression of human sexuality. I counseled her about the risk of sexually transmitted infections during noncoital sexual activity and encouraged efforts to prevent such infections by using condoms during anal–genital intercourse. I also advised sufficient lubrication to avoid any tearing or discomfort. Then I brought the conversation around to Norma's own comfort level with having anal intercourse and emphasized her right to choose. I stressed that anal intercourse was not obligatory, and she need not feel coerced into any sexual activity she did not want.*
>
> *I thought we were finished with questions, but Norma went on to ask, "Well, what about the G-spot?" She and her new partner had been unable to find her G-spot, and Norma was wondering if something was wrong with her. Norma reported that the internet clearly describes an orgasmic area located inside the vagina, about two inches up from the pubic bone on the inner, upper vaginal wall. Again, that gave me pause because I could not give an informed response. I told Norma I needed to do my homework and would talk with her about the G-spot at her next appointment.*
>
> *The G-spot was not covered in my anatomy text nor discussed in any other courses in medical school. I wondered whether an anatomical G-spot actually exists. I certainly had coached women on clitoral orgasm but not a G-spot orgasm. Yet, the G-spot has been in the lay conversation for at least seven decades. Is it myth or reality?*

The G-spot was named for a German scientist, Ernst Gräfenberg, who in 1950 described "an erotic zone located on the anterior wall of the vagina along the course of the urethra that would swell during sexual stimulation." In 1982, Beverly Whipple popularized the G-spot with her book, *The G Spot and Other Discoveries About Human Sexuality.*[5]

The current literature cites dozens of research trials in which the majority of women said they believe a G-spot exists, although not all these women were able to locate it within their own bodies. Objective measures have failed to provide compelling evidence for the existence of a specific anatomical site that could be named the G-spot. Nonetheless, in our conversations with a number of women and men, most believe in the existence of a G-spot. In *The Ultimate Guide to Sex After 50*, Joan Price clearly references the G-spot as a region inside the vagina that can afford great pleasure when stimulated.[6]

> *During our next visit, I told Norma that although many people believe there is a G-spot, science cannot identify a specific anatomical structure that is present in all women. I encouraged Norma to experience orgasms in ways that work for her rather than focusing on something that might not exist. The most important takeaway is this: women have enormous potential to experience orgasms from one or more sources of sensory input.*

Urinary incontinence: Another common issue among postmenopausal women is urinary incontinence—the involuntary leakage of urine. Just as reduced levels of estrogen can cause thinning of the vaginal lining, they can also cause thinning of the lining of the urethra, the tube that passes urine from the bladder out of the body. The surrounding pelvic muscles also may weaken with aging, a process known as pelvic relaxation. Stress incontinence can be the result, and women can have a mix of both stress and urge incontinence.

URINARY INCONTINENCE

Stress incontinence is caused by weak pelvic floor muscles. The most common symptom is leakage of urine with coughing, laughing, sneezing, or lifting objects. Stress incontinence is common during perimenopause but typically doesn't worsen because of menopause.

Urge incontinence (also called *overactive bladder*) is caused by overly active or irritated bladder muscles. The most common symptom is the frequent and sudden urge to urinate, with occasional leakage of urine. Urge incontinence can worsen with age.

Sex is one area in which urinary incontinence can prove troubling. Urinary leakage during intercourse is estimated to affect up to a quarter of women with incontinence. This can be embarrassing for women and lead them to avoid intercourse or to worry about leakage to the point that they are unable to relax and enjoy sex.

NOURISHMENT

Communication—Let's Talk Sex!

Whether the conversations are with your health practitioner, partner, a friend, or sexual counselor, getting your sexual concerns out in the open is the first step. You might ask, "How is communication an integrative strategy?" When it comes to sexual health, it is number one. Much can be done to help women improve their sexual health as they age. We already have shared stories and discussed some treatment strategies.

Now we want to reinforce the need to talk with your partner. Too often women say things like: "We just don't talk about it. We've been married 40 years and have never discussed our sex life. I don't know how I would bring it up. It is just not that important to me." It can be hard to start a conversation about something as personal and intimate as sexuality. Here comes the self-advocacy factor again. We encourage women to start the conversation with their partner if they feel safe and think their partner is approachable. It's essential to avoid any blame or judgment. For example, saying "My doctor wanted me to ask you why we don't have sex" is likely to elicit a defensive, negative response. A better approach might be something like, "I saw my doctor today, and she's writing a book about sexual health in postmenopausal women. She suggested that we might improve our sex life by talking about what we think and asking questions. Are you OK with our sex life?" Of course, your partner's response determines where the conversation goes from there. Sexual performance for many men is a touchy subject, but one that needs to be explored in a relationship. Sometimes the conversation is best done with help from a sex counselor or therapist.

Taking responsibility for your own participation in the sexual dialogue is essential. For instance, if you have low libido or minimal interest, addressing this with your partner is important. You can say, "My doctor told me it is common for women to have a low libido as they age, and that is now true for me." Or, "I wish I had more interest, but I simply don't think about sex. How is that affecting you?" Don't be shy about advocating for a more dynamic sex life with your partner. You could suggest planning a scheduled time to have some sort of intimacy or sexual activity. You might start with once a week or even once a month, depending on what feels reasonable and comfortable. Help create opportunities to discuss ways to enhance your libido and orgasms.

Sex Toys and Self-Pleasuring

Taking a trip to a local sex shop with your partner, where you can peruse different lubricants and various vibrators and sex toys, can be a fun way to open up the conversation about ways to enhance your sexual experience. Most communities have a reputable store where it feels comfortable to browse. Many websites offer online shopping for products that enhance sexual activity and build confidence. Another way to learn about products is through home-hosted parties.

Sex toys, such as vibrators, certainly can add to a woman's ability to orgasm or enhance sensations that are difficult to experience with your own hands or with a partner. Self-exploration opens you up to finding erogenous zones without feeling pressured to please a partner. Or if you do not have a partner, it allows you freedom to pleasure yourself. A guest on the podcast *Woman Over 70: Aging Reimagined* discusses how important masturbation, vibrators, and other sex toys are to maintain a healthy sex life as you age (episode #77).

Hormone Options

Vaginal estrogen is a miracle for a dry vagina when a lubricant is not enough. It is too often underprescribed, either because physicians don't discuss vaginal health with their patients or because they are fearful that it poses health risks. One reason for misperceptions regarding the safety of vaginal estrogen stems from the FDA-issued black-box warning that is on the label of every commercially available vaginal estrogen product. This warning is misleading because it pertains to systemic hormone therapy and not to vaginal estrogen.

> *A friend of mine in her late-60s, who in her younger years had been very sexually active, had not had intercourse since her last relationship 7 years ago. On an excursion to South America, she met a charming younger local man who showed interest in her. She consented to a long weekend away with him, fully intending a sexual rendezvous. In anticipation of having intercourse, she picked up a small supply of lubrication. What she didn't realize was that, unlike in the past, intercourse now would be excruciatingly painful for her. The lubricant was of barely any help. However, the sexual encounter overall aroused such intense feelings of both body and spirit that she continued to have repeated intercourse. It was a memorable, pleasure-filled experience, yet accompanied with considerable vaginal pain. Why was she so unaware of how her dormant vagina would respond? With good humor, my friend tells this story about "the time I neglected to prep my vagina." Lesson learned: prep with vaginal estrogen before adventuring out on a sensuous weekend if you are a postmenopausal woman with an inactive vagina.*

Is vaginal estrogen safe for postmenopausal women? Yes! Please use it if you need it! Most women can use vaginal estrogen with little risk to their system. Even women with a history of breast cancer can use low-dose vaginal estrogen, once risks and benefits have been discussed. Between the years 1982–2012, the Nurses' Health Study investigated the health effects of vaginal estrogen on registered nurses. An important finding was that the use of vaginal estrogen was not associated with a higher risk of cardiovascular disease or cancer.[7]

Low-dose vaginal estrogen therapy is the preferred and *most effective treatment* for genitourinary syndrome of menopause. It is recommended by multiple professional societies, including the North American Menopause Society, the American College of Obstetricians and Gynecologists, and the Endocrine Society.

Vaginal estrogens come in a variety of formulations, including creams and tablets/inserts/suppositories. *Vaginal creams* such as Estrace or Premarin are commercially available; also, compounding pharmacies make less expensive formulations of estradiol (E2) and estriol (E3). An added benefit of the compounding product is you can get one that is hypoallergenic. Creams are beneficial because they can be applied intravaginally and can also be used on the vulva area if it is dry and irritated. Many women also apply a small amount of cream around the urethra if this is contributing to urinary irritation and frequency. The drawbacks of vaginal cream are that some women find it "messy" and/or don't like the feeling of wetness in the vulva area.

Vaginal Estrogen Options

Creams
- Estrace (estradiol)
- Premarin (conjugated estrogen)
- Estradiol (E2) and estriol (E3) from compounding pharmacy

Tablets/Inserts
- Vagifem (estradiol tablet)
- Imvexxy (estradiol insert)
- Estring (estradiol ring)

Vaginal tablets/inserts are another option. Simply placing a tablet or suppository into the vagina is very convenient and less messy than a cream. The tablets/inserts come in lower-dose formulas if you want to minimize estrogen exposure.

If estrogen is prescribed for painful intercourse, dosing of the cream or a tablet starts with nightly use for 2–3 weeks. Once the tissue is restored to a healthier state and intercourse is no longer painful, the dose can be reduced to two times a week. This maintenance therapy is often required to keep the vaginal tissues healthy. If estrogen cream is needed to support vaginal and clitoral tissue for masturbation, then less frequent application may be adequate. Individual women's needs will vary, but some level of estrogen therapy is likely necessary.

The estrogen *vaginal ring* is another way to improve vaginal health. It is placed into the vagina for 3 months. Estradiol is released from the ring on a continuous basis and provides the highest dose of all the commercially available products. This method is very convenient and improves the quality of life for women suffering with significant vaginal dryness/atrophy. The biggest negative is the cost, currently $500 for 3 months, and it is often not covered by insurance. Given likely out-of-pocket expenses, you could use compounding pharmacies for vaginal estradiol (E2) or estriol (E3) creams. Many compounding pharmacies (not FDA approved) will make up a vaginal cream that has the same product as a commercially available estrogen but costs up to two-thirds less and often has fewer chemical additives.

Orgasms are likely to improve once the vagina, vulva, and urethra are healthy with adequate lubrication or with the use of estrogen. With the addition of a good vibrator and a willing partner, you will likely find orgasms come easier. If low libido continues to be a problem, then considering testosterone may be an option.

Testosterone: It's not just men who have the predominant sex hormone testosterone. Women have it, too, although at much lower levels. An individual's testosterone level depends on age, sex, and health. In women, the ovaries produce most of the testosterone with a small amount produced in the adrenal glands. Unfortunately, there are few studies on the role of testosterone deficiency in aging women. However, we do know that, just like in men, testosterone levels in women decline with aging. By age 40, most women's testosterone levels have declined by half, compared to when they were 20.

When low libido persists, despite the aforementioned interventions, testosterone cream can be prescribed. Be aware that testosterone therapy for women is not approved by the FDA, meaning that it is used "off-label." Testosterone is often provided as a compounded topical cream or as a reduced dose of a testosterone gel that is FDA approved for men (eg, AndroGel® 1%).

Myths and misconceptions abound concerning the use of testosterone for women. A common assumption is that testosterone is a "male hormone" and not considered relevant to women. However, quantitatively, testosterone is the most abundant active sex steroid in women throughout their lifespan. It plays an important role in many aspects of a woman's life, not just benefiting sexual drive but also supporting mood (anxiety, irritability, depression), general well-being, physical stamina, muscles, and cognition. Among the fears around testosterone are that it may cause acne, deepening of the voice, growth of hair on the face and chest, lower HDL ("good") cholesterol levels, and male-pattern baldness. Women's responses to testosterone are variable, so proceed cautiously.

> When prescribing testosterone, I start with a low dose, such as 2–5 mg applied topically to the inner thigh. If libido does not improve in 2 weeks, I will double the dose. If after 2 additional weeks, there is still no improvement, I will discontinue treatment. Typically, I will not prescribe more than 10 mg. In cases when the patient's libido improves, I will continue with that dose for 3 months and then check the testosterone level to make sure the levels are not too high.

Many women's health practitioners would welcome a convenient low-dose FDA-approved testosterone product for use in women for sexual health. Currently there are out-of-pocket clinics that are promoting the use of higher-dose testosterone in the form of subcutaneous implant of pellets and intramuscular injections. The concern with these formulations is that the dose can be too high, and once inserted or injected, the testosterone can't be removed. *Regardless of what path is taken, it is important to recognize that there is no testosterone level that will guarantee a satisfactory sex life.*

Pelvic Floor Physical Therapy

Pelvic floor physical therapy involves biofeedback and exercises to encourage relaxation and strengthening of the muscles of the lower pelvis. It purports significant benefits, including improving some forms of urinary incontinence, increasing strength and awareness of the muscles involved in pleasurable sexual sensations, reducing vaginal or pelvic pain during sex, and preventing or treating pelvic organ prolapse (a condition in which the uterus or bladder bulges into the vagina). Pelvic floor physical therapy has helped address sexual problems by improving chronic vaginal or pelvic pain and urinary incontinence.

In a pelvic floor physical therapy session, the physical therapist places biofeedback sensors on the vaginal wall to measure muscle tone and the strength of muscle contractions, which are printed out on a machine. After practicing your exercises at home, you can see your improvement on the machine in your next session. Sometimes the therapist will use a massage-like technique called "myofascial release" to help stretch and release the connective tissue between the skin and the muscles and bones in your pelvic region. Typically, several months of therapy are needed to achieve satisfactory results.

Pelvic floor physical therapy also includes Kegel exercises. "Kegels," as they are commonly called, involve contracting and relaxing the muscles of your pelvic floor, which holds your uterus and bladder in place above your vagina. The key to doing Kegels is identifying the right muscles to contract and relax. If you can stop urinating mid-stream, you've identified the basic move. A couple of tips are to always try to do Kegels when your bladder is empty, and aim to hold your contractions for 2–3 seconds and then release. Once you have the hang of it, do five sets of ten repetitions every day. You can do these while performing routine tasks, such as driving or sitting at your desk. If you have trouble with the technique, ask your physician for a referral to a pelvic floor physical therapist.

HEALING SYSTEMS

Acupuncture/Traditional Chinese Medicine

Seeking out an acupuncturist may not be top of mind when looking for ways to improve your sexual health. You might assume that issues such as low libido or difficulty having an orgasm are strictly related to sexual function or sex organs. In reality, sexual health is a complex intersection of biological, psychological, spiritual, and other factors. A more holistic interpretation from traditional Chinese medicine (TCM) is known as "heart yin deficiency" and "kidney qi deficiency." These deficiencies and other imbalances may interfere with your sexual pleasure. Some people believe that TCM may be better than Western medicine in addressing these complexities. In fact, acupuncture is one of the most common treatments used in TCM to help improve a woman's sexual health by restoring and rebalancing qi. A healthy body and a vibrant sex life emerge when all your parts work in harmony.

Acupuncture needles aim to remove blockages or imbalances in the qi energy that connects the various organs, thereby helping life force and sexual energy to flow. Although there's little research on acupuncture and sexual health, one small study of 35 men and women with sexual dysfunction, likely caused by the antidepressants they were taking for their anxiety or other mood disorders, is intriguing. Patients had nine sessions (15 minutes each) of acupuncture to specifically address "conditions that often included sexual dysfunction." By the end of the study, women reported improved libidos.[8] So, if you are struggling with sexual dysfunction, consider including acupuncture in your wellness web.

Yoga

Yoga can improve women's sexual function? Yes! In fact, some poses specifically strengthen the pelvic and abdominal muscles. The potential sexual benefits may result from yoga's relaxing effects, the pelvis-strengthening effects of many poses, and focusing attention on sensation. In one study of sexually active women ages 22–55, the women completed a sexual function questionnaire before and after a 12-week yoga program. Each day, women practiced yoga for an hour, followed by breathing and relaxation exercises. The before and after self-reports showed improved sexual function scores in all six areas studied: desire, arousal, lubrication, orgasm, satisfaction, and pain. In fact, 75% of the women reported that their sex lives had improved, with the biggest improvements seen in women 45 and older.

Two specific yoga poses you can try to help are the happy baby and the chair pose.

> *Happy baby* pose allows the pelvic floor to stretch maximally. Lie on your back, and, as you inhale, bend your knees and bring them toward your chest. Open your knees wide, bringing them toward your armpits. Your shins should be perpendicular to the floor, with your ankles in line with your knees. Grab the outside edges of your feet, and gently push your feet up into your hands while pulling back with your arms.
>
> *Chair pose* is really good for the pelvic floor, which is stretched when going down, and lifted when coming up. Start in mountain pose, with your arms out in front of you, parallel to the floor. Bend your knees and push your hips back in a squat, as if you were going to sit into a chair. Keep your hips higher than your knees.

Kundalini yoga is a spiritual and physical practice that combines movement, breath, meditation, and chanting. Kundal, derived from the Sanskrit "coiled energy," refers to energy gathered at the base of your spine that needs to be released. Many of the repetitive postures help move the energy and strengthen pelvic muscles, which can enhance sexual energy.

Some of you are familiar with the *Kama Sutra*, the ancient Sanskrit text that, over the years, has become the go-to guide for intricate sex positions. You don't have to do overtly sexual, Kama Sutra–style poses if this seems too much. Instead, do regular yoga poses that relax you, loosen the pelvic area, boost your mood, and heighten your sexual desire.

Remember that you need to pay attention to your sexual health (self), including the health of your vagina, just like you need to pay attention to the health of all the other parts of your body. You may want to consider some of these integrative strategies to improve your sexual health and well-being.

PATHWAYS TO ENERGIZE FLOW

> **Self-Awareness:** What are your sensual and sexual pleasures? How do you feel about the presence or absence of sexual activity in your life?
>
> **Self-Compassion:** Give yourself permission to give and receive simple acts of loving-kindness. Claim yourself as a sexual being.
>
> **Self-Advocacy:** What might you explore to enhance your sexual health? With whom do you want to communicate your needs?

CATHERINE'S PATHWAY

This is an awkward topic for me to talk about so publicly, yet I think it's important that we aging women take stock of our sexual health and be open about it.

I am a 72-year-old heterosexual woman who enjoys sex and am currently without a steady sexual partner. Perhaps like some of you, I know about the "use-it-or-lose-it" nature of the vagina. I am grateful that I have always been comfortable with self-pleasuring. Vibrators are good—wish I could purchase one of Grace and Frankie's *(television series). Yet, I miss the intimacy of touch with another person.*

Friends and I fret a bit about our physical changes—bulges in the wrong places, saggy upper arms, and droopy breasts. We wonder about feeling sexually attractive in our aging bodies. And then we say, "yes"; our bodies are primed for sensual pleasure.

In spite of horror stories I hear from women about their online dating experiences, I might try that this year . . . or next (hardly a firm commitment). I will commit to a regular routine of body work that involves touch. I am curious about Kundalini yoga as a means to enhance sexual energy. And I will continue to talk openly about sexual health with my friends—how we feel about our needs and wants, and what we envision for our future.

6 Sleep
Create Your Rhythm

Do you have difficulty getting to sleep, experience frequent waking during the night, or have early morning wakefulness? Sleep disruption is so prevalent that up to 60% of postmenopausal women can identify with this struggle. "I just can't sleep." "I only get real sleep two hours a night. I can't go on like this." "What I wouldn't give for a good night's sleep!"

According to the study of Women's Health Across the Nation, sleep disturbance increases with advancing age and significantly affects our health and well-being.[1] The most common sleep disruption in women is difficulty getting to sleep, which correlates strongly with anxiety and ruminating thoughts. The second most common disruption is waking to go to the bathroom, which most older women have to do at least once during the night. Once up to urinate, many women have difficulty getting back to sleep, and the disruptive sleep patterns continue.

It's no surprise that we often don't sleep well as we age. You might have been told that older people don't need as much sleep as when they were younger adults, but that notion is not supported by the research. We still need the same amount of sleep, about 8 hours every night, although some women seem to do well on less. Among the myriad factors that might be causing your sleep disturbances are normal physiological changes associated with aging, poor sleep hygiene, menopausal-like symptoms, urinary frequency, mood disorders, chronic pain or other health issues, and disruptions in your external environment. Some women suffer from sleep disorders like obstructive sleep apnea and restless leg syndrome.

UNDERSTANDING SLEEP

The reality is that sleep is complicated, so let's try to better understand the nature of sleep problems. Three different yet interrelated sleep problems, often lumped together as insomnia, are sleep deprivation, acute insomnia, and chronic insomnia.

Sleep deprivation is a common problem if you are shortening your sleep time by choice or out of habit. In this age of technology, you have more choices for things to do late at night. Many experts believe that people today are overstimulated, unable to settle their minds and focus on rest. In the past, people used to wind down in the evening with relaxing activities such as reading, evening devotions, and simple card games. But now, we can easily be wound up by television, mobile devices, computers, and the list goes on. Consequently, your normal biorhythm becomes disrupted.

DOI: 10.1201/9781003250968-8

Insomnia is the inability to sleep even when you give yourself the opportunity for sleep. Approximately 60 million Americans suffer from insomnia, which is categorized as either acute/episodic or chronic.

Acute or episodic insomnia affects 30% of the population at some point in their lives. These episodic sleepless nights typically last for less than 3 months and often are related in time to an identifiable cause.

Chronic insomnia affects 5% of the population. The person's sleep system has gone awry—it's in a state of disrepair and has stopped functioning properly. Chronic insomnia can have a major negative impact on your quality of life and health, and it needs to be treated.

CIRCADIAN RHYTHM

Circadian rhythm is basically a 24-hour internal clock that runs in the background of your brain and cycles between sleepiness and alertness at regular intervals.

In *Why We Sleep*, Matthew Walker makes sense of sleep from a biochemical model.[2] If you really want to understand sleep, this is an excellent book on the subject. He describes the circadian rhythm, which is essential to sleeping well, as well as another principle called "sleep pressure." This latter phenomenon is created by a chemical called adenosine building up in your brain. Adenosine is like a barometer that registers the amount of time that has elapsed since waking. Adenosine rises throughout the day, and, when it peaks, it signals a strong desire to sleep. This sleep pressure phenomenon happens to most people after they've been up for 12–16 hours. If you listen to this signal and go to bed when cued, your sleep will improve. Walker's perspective is that sleep represents overnight therapy and that we should "give in to sleep" rather than mandate it. However, the sleep pressure signal of adenosine is easily muted by using stimulants such as caffeine or simply resisting the urge to sleep. And this is exactly what many of us do to get our work done or participate in social events. But we pay a price—ignoring sleep pressure will eventually throw off our circadian rhythm.

WHY IS SLEEP SO IMPORTANT?

Your sleep is as important as your waking hours, and you should value it. Sleep is an essential function that allows your body and mind to recharge, leaving you refreshed and alert when you wake up. The consequences of sleep deprivation are serious and can lead to poorer mental functioning, lack of attention, a distorted sense of time, and daytime fatigue. In *Keep Smart*, Dr. Sanjay Gupta points out that sleep has protective benefits for the brain. He describes that during sleep there is a sort of "rinse cycle" in which certain neurotrophic factors bathe the brain and help remove toxic waste products.[3]

BRIDGING THE GAP

Some women with insomnia are helped considerably with low-dose, tricyclic-related medications, such as trazodone or mirtazapine. While these medications are relatively safe and nonaddictive, dependency can build up. Other medications that are sedatives/ hypnotics, such as zolpidem (Ambien), are preferred by some women because they help induce sleep and allow one to wake up feeling well rested without any hangover effect. Another class of drugs called benzodiazepines, such as lorazepam (Ativan) and alprazolam (Xanax), are commonly used but are best avoided on a nightly basis because of their addictive potential. The problem is that once you start taking a drug like Ambien, it's hard to "give it up" because it works so well. But you may not realize there are many subtle side effects, such as increased risk of mild dementia and decreased cognition. Once you reach age 70, Ambien becomes less appealing because it increases the risk of falling and is also unlikely to be covered by insurance.

> *Elaine, age 76, struggled with chronic anxiety and insomnia. Yoga and a regular meditation practice helped considerably with managing her anxiety, but her sleeping difficulty persisted. Sometime during her 60s, she started occasionally using Ambien for sleep, but eventually she was taking 10 mg every night. I saw her fairly often and always discouraged her nightly use of Ambien, although I continued to prescribe it for her, managing to decrease her dose to 5 mg. Over time, I noticed that her memory was not as good and word finding was more difficult. I became more concerned and referred Elaine for a neuropsych evaluation. The results came back relatively normal. Elaine's husband accompanied her on a follow-up visit as he, too, was noticing some changes in her memory. With notepad in hand, he eagerly wrote down my recommendations for his wife. While Elaine was talking to me, she had a sudden lapse of consciousness. Although she seemed alert, she answered my questions with either a vague response or just a blank stare. Her husband and I shared concerned looks, and I knew there was a problem. It looked as though Elaine might be having a stroke or other neurologic event right in front of our eyes.*
>
> *Elaine was quickly transported to the emergency room for immediate attention. After a thorough evaluation with brain scans, EEGs, and lab testing, over 3 days of hospitalization, nothing was clearly identified. When Elaine returned to her baseline status, she was discharged with the explanation for the episode likely being the use of Ambien. Over the next 2 months, she gradually weaned down the dose from 5 mg to 0.5 mg, yet her sleep remained disruptive, despite a regular sleep schedule and good sleep hygiene. Elaine and her husband were determined to get her off Ambien, even though it had worked far better than other sleep medications she had tried. Finally, with the help of a low-dose tricyclic antidepressant, she was successful. Once off the Ambien, Elaine's memory and word-finding skills noticeably improved.*

Elaine's story serves to remind women with chronic insomnia that as hard as it may be to avoid Ambien because you feel desperate, don't use it on a nightly basis. You will likely become dependent on it. It doesn't resolve the underlying problem and likely contributes to other problems.

INTEGRATIVE STRATEGIES

You must learn to recognize your own innate circadian rhythms and how to address common sleep challenges. "Sleep is a non-negotiable pillar of well-being." This is the advice of integrative psychiatrist Dr. Henry Emmons, whose books, *Chemistry of Joy* and *Chemistry of Calm*, are excellent sources of information on depression and anxiety.[4–5] Sleep is the central lifestyle measure for the brain, mood, and overall health. It is one of the main requirements for recovering fully from depression, anxiety, or other illnesses.

HORMONE THERAPY

The hot flashes and night sweats that are so common during and after menopause clearly exacerbate sleep changes. A trial of hormone therapy may be warranted to see if sleep improves, with a subsequent improvement of mood, memory, and fatigue. This choice should be made through shared decision-making with your health practitioner.

Estrogen: Estrogen therapy, with or without progesterone, is very effective in treating vasomotor symptoms and decreasing frequent nighttime awakenings.

Progesterone: Studies have shown that decreases in progesterone levels can cause disturbed sleep. Progesterone has both sedative and anxiolytic effects, and prescription of progesterone alone is reasonable if sleep disruption and fatigue are the only complaints and night sweats seem minimal.

HOLISTIC SLEEP HYGIENE

Practicing good sleep hygiene is essential for optimal sleep. Considerable research has gone into developing a set of guidelines and tips for improving sleep quality. Evidence suggests that these strategies can provide long-term solutions to sleep difficulties. However, many people are resistant to the idea of sleep hygiene. Why is it that sleep hygiene is so easily dismissed? Probably it's because we enjoy habits that prevent optimal sleep. For example, you may like reading in bed, going on Facebook, answering a few emails, playing games on your smartphone, or going to bed whenever you feel like it. This is another example of *immunity to change* (discussed in Chapter 3). If you struggle with chronic insomnia, then changing these behaviors is in your best interest. Following simple sleep hygiene techniques will greatly benefit your well-being.

SLEEP STRATEGIES

- Keep the bedroom cool (65 degrees is optimal).
- Keep the bedroom dark (the darker, the better).
- Keep the bedroom quiet (the quieter, the better).
- Relax your mind and body.
- Go to bed at the same time every night.
- Get up at the same time every day.
- Do not read or watch television in bed.
- Do not eat, drink alcohol, or exercise before bedtime.
- Avoid screen (computer, phone, television) exposures for at least 1 hour before bedtime.

Think of sleep as a restorative, life-giving act. Commit to creating a sacred space reserved for only sleep and sex. Keep a routine, going to bed and getting up at more or less the same time every day, even on weekends and days off. If you have a bad night's sleep and are tired, it is important to try and keep your daytime activities the same as you had planned. Don't avoid activities because you feel tired, because this can reinforce insomnia.

Avoid using alcohol to help you get to sleep. Likely, you will wake after a few hours and be unable to get back to sleep. When you have a glass or two of wine before bed, your blood sugar rises, resulting in a surge of insulin that is then followed by a drop in blood sugar levels. Your body perceives this as stressful, and you wake up. Simple dietary changes such as avoiding alcohol late in the evening and reducing caffeine and sugar consumption often improve sleep quality and reduce daytime fatigue.

Relax before bedtime. Take a warm bath, drink herbal tea, or listen to a soothing audio recording. This strategy cannot be emphasized enough, even though it is often minimized and dismissed. Keep your room cool and make sure your bedroom is dark with no television, no laptop, no smartphone, and no electronic magnetic field (EMF) exposure.

Studies show that playing computer games affects the amount of time it takes to fall asleep and the amount of rapid eye movement sleep. There is also public concern about sleep disturbances due to radiofrequency-EMF exposure. A few small studies suggest that EMFs can impede the production of melatonin and affect the body's circadian rhythm, thereby undermining the sleep cycle. Another major concern is that EMFs have the potential to interfere with how cells in the body communicate with one another, inhibit the cells' ability to detoxify and repair themselves, and disrupt our subtle electromagnetic systems. With the onslaught of strong EMF exposure in recent decades because of technological devices, the potential effects are not yet clear, and it may take some time before we know the consequences. In the meantime, some pointers include turning off your cell phone, replacing cordless phones in your bedroom with a wired (landline) phone, and removing wireless speakers from the bedroom (these also emit EMFs).

Carolyn has heard many stories from women who claim much improved sleep and improved well-being after eliminating EMFs in the bedroom. One woman in particular stands out because she was not a typical seeker of integrative medicine.

Agnes, age 80, had been a primary care patient of mine for years. She was extremely active, working full-time as a nurse supervisor at a local assisted-living facility. She loved her job and worked long hours into the evening, coming home exhausted and ready for sleep. She did not have a history of sleep problem but started to have difficulty falling to sleep. One day, an electrician doing a job in her home mentioned that she should remove her television and smartphone from the bedroom. He told her about the increased exposure to EMFs and possible harmful effects on sleep and general health. Agnes had never heard of EMF exposure but thought, "I'll give it a try. I'm not sleeping, so what have I got to lose?" She removed the television from the bedroom, as well as the jacks for the phone and computer. Much to her surprise and relief, her sleep improved immediately. At first, I thought Agnes was benefiting from a placebo effect, but 6 months later, she was still reporting good sleep and avoiding wireless devices in her bedroom.

Removing these devices from your bedroom is a good practice to consider. Reducing your EMF exposure is a way to take back your environment in a positive and life-centric way. If you are interested in knowing your exposure to EMFs, you can look for an EMF practitioner who will come to your home and/or workplace to measure the level of EMFs in the environment.

Research is ongoing about potential negative health effects from high exposures to EMFs. For more information on this subject, consider listening to Devra Davis, *5G, Wireless Radiation and Health: A Scientific and Policy Update (2020) on* YouTube or listen to YouTube videos by Shield Your Body. The last thing we want to do is promote false narratives or conspiracy theories that create doubt about the value of science, yet we remain open about potential environmental harm that needs to be researched for safety.

NOURISHMENT

Supplements

Magnesium is the first supplement to try if you are having trouble with sleep. Magnesium is just part of the story for better sleep, but some women respond remarkably well. Magnesium is most effective when used in conjunction with sleep hygiene measures. If you think that taking magnesium at night is going to be the magic bullet without changing some of your bad sleep habits, you will be disappointed. However, if you create an environment that is conducive to sleep, avoid those electronic devices, and spend some time relaxing and preparing for a restful sleep, the addition of magnesium can help calm your muscles and your mind.

Magnesium is an essential mineral that plays an important role in many biological functions, including nerve and muscle function. Older people tend to have lower levels of magnesium than younger adults. A complicating factor is that certain medications often taken by aging women, such as hydrochlorothiazide (a diuretic) or proton-pump inhibitors (eg, omeprazole), can interfere with magnesium absorption.

A popular product used by women is "Calm," a highly absorbable blend of magnesium citrate when combined with water. A half-hour before bedtime, drink a cup of warm water with a teaspoon of powder (205 mg) mixed in. Magnesium is also available in pill form; the most effective dose is typically 200–400 mg. Another product, magnesium glycinate (240–360 mg), is a gentle form of magnesium for women sensitive to magnesium citrate or oxide because it is less likely to have a laxative effect.

Epsom salts are a form of magnesium sulfate. Epsom salt baths are a longtime home remedy and can help with muscle relaxation before bedtime. Even just soaking your feet in an Epsom salt and warm water solution can help relax you before going to bed.

L-tryptophan is an amino acid that is used to support restful sleep. Tryptophan is an essential amino acid, meaning the body cannot synthesize it; it must be obtained from the diet. Once in the brain, tryptophan is converted to serotonin, which is further metabolized into melatonin by the pineal gland. Evidence indicates that L-tryptophan

MAGNESIUM OPTIONS

Magnesium citrate is one of the most popular and easily absorbed magnesium supplements. This form of magnesium binds to citric acid, which is a mild laxative. So, magnesium citrate is a good choice for individuals with occasional constipation.

Magnesium oxide is one of the least absorbed forms of magnesium, but it delivers one of the highest percentages of elemental magnesium per dose. This makes it a good choice for someone who wants to take as few capsules as possible. Like magnesium citrate, magnesium oxide can be helpful for those with occasional constipation.

Magnesium glycinate is a gentle form of magnesium that binds to glycine, a nonessential amino acid that is thought to have relaxing effects. It could be one of the best types of magnesium for those who want to promote mental calm, relaxation, and good quality sleep. It is less likely to have a laxative effect than magnesium oxide or citrate.

Magnesium malate is another gentle form of magnesium that is often recommended for people suffering from fatigue and symptoms of fibromyalgia. Malate is formed when magnesium is attached to malic acid (a compound found in fruit), and it plays a key role in energy production.

in doses of 1 gram or more increases sleepiness and decreases the time it takes to fall sleep. Vitamin B_6 is often added to the formula to provide enhanced support.

Melatonin is a hormone produced by the pineal gland to help set the timing of sleep onset. The circadian rhythm is associated with melatonin release, which is highly synchronized with our habitual hours of sleep and regulates the timing of sleep. Melatonin sends a message to the sleep-generator regions of the brain that it is dark and time to get ready for sleep. Because melatonin levels fall significantly during and after menopause, a trial of melatonin therapy is a very reasonable and safe option to see if sleep improves. As with other supplements, melatonin works best when combined with sleep hygiene strategies and a regular sleep time routine. The usual starting dose is 0.3 mg, which can be increased incrementally up to 5 mg if needed.

L-theanine is a compound found naturally in the tea plant (*Camellia sinensis*). It is thought to promote relaxation and facilitate sleep by contributing to a number of changes in the brain. It boosts levels of neurotransmitters like GABA (gamma-aminobutyric acid), serotonin, and dopamine, and it increases alpha brain wave activity that induces relaxation. Research shows that L-theanine may improve quality of sleep, not by acting as a sedative but by lowering anxiety and promoting relaxation. The recommended dose is 100–400 mg, taken 1–2 hours before bedtime.

It's important to remember that individual women may respond differently to a supplement. While supplements work wonders for many women, others may experience an undesirable side effect. Paying attention to how your body responds to any new medication, supplement, or modality is essential. Consider this cautionary tale about Carolyn's trip to Guatemala in 2018.

> *Before my trip, I had been seeing a therapist to help deal with stress and work-life transition. She suggested that I try magnesium and L-theanine to dampen some of the anxiety and improve my restless sleep. I started the supplement about a week before my travels, and it seemed to be helping. Five days into my trip, I developed a considerable amount of abdominal bloating, and 2 days later, my belly had become a hard, round, bloated drum. I thought maybe I had picked up a gastrointestinal infection from contaminated food or water, but it didn't feel like any GI infection I had experienced during prior travels. When I reflected further to figure out if I had done anything different—bingo! I had been taking magnesium/theanine nightly for the last three weeks! While I really didn't think this benign supplement could be the cause, I decided to stop taking it anyway to see what would happen. Within 24 hours, my abdominal bloating and other symptoms resolved.*

Light Therapy

An effective and safe integrative strategy for improved sleep and diminished daytime somnolence is exposure to full-spectrum bright light in the early morning. Light therapy is especially helpful when the problem is related to circadian rhythm disturbances caused by jet lag or shift work. Bright light effective for therapy means outdoor sunlight or artificial bright indoor lighting (many commercial light devices are available). Normal indoor lighting (about 100 lux) is of insufficient intensity. Research has shown that light needs to be about 1,000 lux or more to be effective at phase changing the circadian rhythm. More recent research also has shown that it is the shorter wavelength light—blue light—that is most effective in changing the timing of the circadian rhythm. To be effective, light needs to enter the eyes; however, staring at the light source is not necessary. You can be eating a meal, watching television, or working on a computer while receiving the light stimulus in your visual field.

Botanicals

Valerian: Valeriana officinalis is a perennial plant native to Europe, Asia, and North America. It has a long history of use in traditional medicine and is often combined with other herbs. Valerian root is most commonly used for its sedative and hypnotic properties in patients with insomnia, and it has a mechanism of action similar to that of benzodiazepines. Research studies suggest that valerian may improve sleep quality, but many of these studies had methodologic problems, limiting firm conclusions. Nevertheless, a trial of valerian in conjunction with good sleep hygiene may be worthwhile. The typical dose for valerian is a 500-mg tablet taken at least 30 minutes before bedtime to prevent any reflux when lying down. The taste is unpleasant, and it is commonly combined with other herbs, including passionflower, hops, and lemon balm.

Lavender: The name *L. angustifolia* is derived from the Latin word *lavare*, which means to wash or bathe. The fragrance from lavender oil is believed to induce a calming and sedentary effect to improve sleep and is used as an aromatherapy.

Single-blind randomized studies have shown that lavender has a positive impact on energy level, sleep quality, and overall well-being. In a 2018 study of 30 nursing home residents, lavender aromatherapy improved the onset, quality, and duration of sleep in this older adult population.[6]

AROMATHERAPY

Aromatherapy uses essential oils, which are highly concentrated substances extracted from flowers, leaves, stalks, fruits, and roots, and distilled from resins. Essential oils are a mixture of saturated and unsaturated hydrocarbons, alcohol, aldehydes, esters, ethers, ketones, oxides, phenols, and terpenes, which may produce characteristic odors.

Using natural remedies like lavender can help to quiet the nervous system before sleep. Different formulations of lavender are used for aromatherapy to assist in sleep, including inhalation, massage, or simple applications on the skin. A newer, convenient formulation of lavender is a patch, which improved sleep in small, randomized studies.

Cognitive Behavior Therapy-Insomnia (CBT-I)

"Sleep boot camp" is what Mary called her treatment protocol.

At age 73, Mary said she hadn't slept well for years. Now, exhausted and wanting to "fix the problems," she agreed to see a behavior sleep therapist who was a psychologist well known for helping many people with chronic insomnia. Mary admitted she had little faith that the program would work because she'd tried everything in the past without success. However, 2 months after starting the program, she was amazed at how well it had worked. She also reported that resetting her circadian rhythm required a time commitment. "I am sleeping, but it is a discipline and, if I get off my routine, my sleep suffers."

CBT-I is a drug-free therapy that seeks to reestablish the patient's sleep process. Initially, the amount of sleep time is reduced as a way to increase sleep drive and retrain the body to sleep normally. This also serves as a method to stop spending time in bed while awake. The goal is to weaken the association between being in bed and having anxiety about not falling asleep.

In 2005, the National Institutes of Health recommended that CBT-I should be the first-line treatment for chronic insomnia, before medications are prescribed. However, a public and professional bias toward the use of medications and the lack of awareness of CBT-I as a newer treatment approach are key factors that have limited progress. Another huge factor is that this therapy is not a quick fix. It takes weeks to shift the circadian rhythm, and patients are often desperate and impatient for results.

Insomnia triggers may be different for each person. Seeing a sleep therapist who is knowledgeable about CBT-I is the first step. Typically, the process of CBT-I involves restricting sleep through phases that occur over several weeks. The purpose of resetting your circadian system is to retrain your brain to have an automatic sleep response that allows you to sustain sleep throughout the night.

> *Marcia developed sleep issues beginning with menopause. Over the course of a few years, sleep became more problematic and interfered with her work commitments. Initially, when she had a few nights when she couldn't get to sleep, she would take Ativan (a benzodiazepine) or Ambien. Eventually, she needed to take either one or the other every night. By age 64, Marcia was determined to get off medication. She already exercised regularly and ate a healthy diet. Her sleep hygiene, on the other hand, was somewhat compromised. She worked late into the evening on her computer, often didn't get into bed until 11 p.m. or later, and then read for a half-hour or so. It was hard for Marcia to break these habits to improve her sleep hygiene, but she was determined to get better sleep. Adding magnesium and melatonin to her nightly routine helped some, but she continued to have nighttime waking. We talked about CBT-I, and Marcia tried a modified program given the time constraints on her life. She forced herself to stay up until 1 a.m. every night until she was so exhausted that she was able to get 6 hours of sleep before getting up for work. Gradually, she was able to move her bedtime to 10:30 p.m., which she was able to maintain by adhering to good sleep hygiene habits.*

HEALING SYSTEMS

Ayurvedic Medicine

Ayurveda is a system of healing that offers a unique self-discovery approach to healthcare. With its roots in ancient India, Ayurveda is a tradition thought to be over 5,000 years old. The name Ayurveda is derived from two words in Sanskrit: *ayur* meaning "life or longevity" and *veda* meaning "science or sacred knowledge." Ayurveda's definition, therefore, roughly translates as "the science of longevity" or "the sacred knowledge of life."

This system is founded on the principle that nature—both within us and in life as a whole—functions through five natural elements: space, air, fire, water, and earth. These five elements in turn constitute three doshas, which are aspects of nature's intelligence. The doshas guide the three fundamental functions required for all life: movement, metabolism, and structure. You have your own dosha or constitution. One source of information to better understand your constitution/dosha is www.banyonbotanicals.com.

> *Vata* governs movement (air and space). It is subtle, light, cool, dry, quick, and variable, and it leads the other doshas.
> *Pitta* governs metabolism and transformation (fire and water). It is the only dosha with heat and is responsible for digestion, metabolism, and energy production.
> *Kapha* governs structure (earth and water). It is heavy, dense, and structural, and it composes the physical, material substance of the body (muscles, bones, and fluids).

While the three doshas of Vata, Pitta, and Kapha are present in everyone, each person has a dominant dosha or a combination of two doshas. When you understand how to balance your doshas, you can dramatically improve your quality of life and ease chronic health problems, especially insomnia. Understanding your constitution, or dosha, and matching your lifestyle accordingly are essential in the Ayurvedic tradition. Consulting with an Ayurvedic practitioner is often the best approach to better understand and benefit from the healing power of Ayurvedic medicine.

> *Judy, a 60-year-old attorney, came into my office because of heartburn and a skin rash around her pant line at the waist. She had been working on a big case and found herself becoming very irritable and unable to sleep. Her partner commented that her shift in behavior was affecting their relationship. Judy had seen an Ayurvedic practitioner in the past and was familiar with Ayurvedic principles. Although I am not an Ayurvedic practitioner, I was able to see by her physical appearance that she had an imbalance in the Pitta dosha with too much fire and heat. I suggested that she cool down her Pitta dosha and balance out her excess fire. She acknowledged that her busy work schedule had kept her out of touch with her body, and she needed a reminder to revisit "cooling" strategies. She agreed that a revisit with her Ayurvedic practitioner was needed, but she could do some self-treatment in the meantime. We discussed the need to slow down and eat three meals, with the biggest meal being at noon, and to take a relaxing cooling bath before bedtime to help improve sleep.*

Essential to Judy getting better sleep was identifying that she had a problem and being willing to make the necessary changes. Often, becoming aware of what is happening in your body and then deciding to make a change is difficult. This again highlights the "immunity to change" approach discussed in Chapter 3.

If you were to look to Ayurvedic practices to guide your sleep, a Kapha quality to the hours of 7 p.m. to 10 p.m. makes you feel heavy and sleepy. If you go to bed early enough to catch that wave, it will ride you right into sleep. Starting around 10 p.m., a Pitta, or fiery energy, takes hold. This can feel like a second wind, and, if you are still awake, you may suddenly want to do projects around the house or mindlessly scan Instagram. One of the best ways to set yourself up for falling asleep more easily and sleeping more efficiently is to get in bed by 10 p.m.

Simple Ayurvedic remedies can help:

Cool foot bath: If you "run hot" in the middle of the night, thoroughly rinse your feet with cool water before bed (and if you wake during the night). Ayurveda connects the feet with the fire element. Cooling down the feet is a time-tested way to refresh the mind and return to restful sleep.

Early supper: Eating a big, late meal demands more of your digestion than it can handle at that time of night, which reduces digestive strength and prevents sound sleep. Ayurveda recommends making lunch the biggest meal of the day (when the Pitta fire of digestion is strongest), eating a light meal around sunset, and allowing at least 2 hours to digest before bedtime.

Reducing alcohol consumption: If you wake in the middle of the night with sweltering feet, night sweats, or hot flashes, the sharp, Pitta-provoking fire of alcohol may not be helping. Alcohol often initially helps people fall asleep, but then overstimulates the liver (a Pitta organ) and causes a restless, fiery body and mind. Reduce or avoid alcohol at night and see how much better you sleep.

Adding weight: If Vata has you feeling restless or fidgety, try putting an extra blanket or pillow on your legs at night. Vata governs the legs, and excess lightness or movement in the legs can disturb sleep. In the same way that using sandbags on the legs helps some people settle into Savasana, putting a little weight on the legs can be a simple, effective way to ground Vata at bedtime.

Self-massage: Both Vata and Pitta are supported by a simple massage before bed. Key areas to rub are the feet, low back, ears, and head. Use slow, soft strokes for Vata, and a bit more vigorous rubbing for Pitta to dilate the blood vessels and release heat. The following seasons are valued in the Ayurvedic tradition. For example, warming sesame oil is best for Vata types and for cooler months, and cooling coconut oil is good for Pitta constitutions or for warmer times of year.

Yoga

We discussed the value of yoga in the previous chapter, and yoga to enhance sleep is yet one more benefit. Yoga postures are designed to help you calm your body, mind, and soul so you can relax and get to sleep with ease. A review and meta-analysis of 19 studies representing nearly 2,000 women with sleep problems found that, overall, a yoga practice at any time of the day improved sleep quality.

Before you try these poses, set the stage for sleep by centering your mind and applying sleep hygiene principles. It helps to alleviate worry and get into a positive mindset to relax. Then try these gentle poses.

Knee hug: If you have back issues and have been sitting all day, the knee hug will feel particularly nourishing and relieve tension. Many of us work hunched over at a desk all day or spend hours on the computer. This can result in tight muscles and limited range of motion.

> *How to:* Lie down and hug one or both knees into your chest. Whether you do one or both depends on your physical abilities. If you can hug both knees into your chest at the same time, rock from side to side to massage your spine.

Shoulder shrug: Holding tension in your neck and shoulders is a common result of working long hours on the computer, staring at your phone, or being in Zoom meetings all day.

> *How to:* Sit straight up on your bed, with good posture. Inhale, bring your shoulders up to your ears, and squeeze your arm and shoulder muscles tightly. Exhale and release your shoulders, pulling your shoulder blades downward. Repeat a few times.

Corpse pose: If you practice yoga, you know this as Savasana, which is often the final pose of most yoga classes. It looks extremely easy to lie down and do nothing, but it's among the hardest poses to master because it requires you to release all physical and emotional tension and let go of mental thoughts. As the thoughts come into your mind, just notice them, acknowledge them, and then let them go.

How to: Lie down with your arms at your sides, palms up and relaxed. Close your eyes and focus on the rise and fall of your breath. If you have trouble with intrusive thoughts, acknowledge their presence and picture them floating away.

Yoga belly breathing: If you can only do one thing to prepare yourself for sleep, take a few minutes to focus on your breath. The abdominal breath, also known as the "yoga belly breath," is helpful. Often women are in the habit of breathing shallowly from the chest, but deeper breaths fill the lungs completely. This triggers a cascade of physiological changes. Your heart rate slows, your blood pressure decreases, and muscle tension eases.

How to: Lying down, put one hand below your belly button. Breathe in through your nose to fill your lungs and pay attention to how your belly rises. Breathe out through your nose, releasing the air into the lungs and flattening the belly. Repeat for a few minutes.

———————

Ayurvedic medicine and yoga are just two of the many healing modalities that can offer a pathway to better sleep. Incorporating holistic sleep hygiene measures into your nighttime routine will offer considerable support to a healthy sleep rhythm. Although we don't know everything there is to know about sleep and all its benefits, we know for sure that we need sleep, not just to survive but to thrive.

PATHWAYS TO CREATE YOUR RHYTHM

Self-Knowing: What changes have you noticed about your sleep patterns? Might some of your habits be getting in the way of a good night sleep?

Self-Compassion: You know your body needs sleep. Value your sleep as much as you value your waking hours.

Self-Advocacy: How can you reclaim your right to a good night sleep? What are you willing to do to make sleep a restorative practice?

———————

CATHERINE'S PATHWAY

Before menopause, I had an enviable talent for getting a good night's sleep. I could fall asleep, stay asleep, and wake refreshed. But after menopause, sleeping well became a constant challenge. I need at least 7–8 hours to function at my best. I value sleep as much as waking hours, and I'll do what it takes to get it. A rather dramatic example is that I took Ambien nightly for 12 years. Various doctors— primary physician, sleep expert, gynecologist, oncologist—had all okayed staying on Ambien because it worked so well for me, even after reducing the dose from 10 to 5 mg. Why then, at age 70, did I get off Ambien? First of all, my health insurance would no longer cover Ambien after age 70. As I was exploring other options, my primary physician prescribed trazodone to help with sleep during healing from shingles and back pain. I stopped Ambien cold turkey and have enjoyed relatively restful sleep with trazodone, a nonaddictive option, ever since.

Since working on this chapter, I have become more intentional about using natural strategies to support my sleep. I aim for a light supper, earlier in the evening. With regard to my red wine habit, I limit the intake (usually) and stop a bit before bedtime (usually). Also, before bedtime, typically around 10 p.m., I've added magnesium as a supplement. Once in the bedroom, which I do keep cool and dark, I try to not watch television, except on occasion. I really don't want to break the delicious habit of reading before falling asleep. So, if my reading overstimulates me, I practice deep breathing exercises and have lavender aromatherapy on hand.

7 Anxiety
Calm Your Mind

If anxiety is a familiar feeling, you are certainly not alone. Unfortunately, many women suffer in silence believing no one will understand how worry, fear, and anxious thoughts can overwhelm their daily life. For this reason, we have included anxiety among the eight health conditions that are common to postmenopausal women. You may ask, "Isn't anxiety just all in your mind?" No, it is not. Anxiety is an emotional, mental, and physical phenomenon closely associated with menopause and postmenopause.

Are you aware that two-thirds of adults who deal with anxiety are women? As a postmenopausal woman, you are at even higher risk. This is because the shifts in your hormonal landscape can affect how your brain responds to stressors. With aging, you may be more vulnerable to an anxious state as you face new stressors: health challenges, change in professional standing and other identities, uncertain living situations, financial concerns, and loss of partners and friends. So, it's possible that anxiety, even if it was not bothersome to you before menopause, could be a new occurrence. Or, if you are quite familiar with anxiety, it could escalate with more or different life stressors. Even if anxiety is not part of your experience, you very likely have a family member or friend who is dealing with it.

You may know anxiety as a feeling of unease, tension, nervousness, and/or worry. Almost everyone experiences these feelings in various times and circumstances. Anxiety is a normal response to something that is not right. It signals you to pay attention to the situation. Anxious feelings can help focus your mind as you navigate the various forces and stressors of everyday, postmenopausal life. However, if the feelings of unease and worry accompany you everywhere, through many situations, then you might have an actual anxiety disorder. This shows up as excessive and persistent worry, tension, and nervousness, often with physical symptoms. You may not be aware of how much of your time and energy is consumed by worry and how long you've been holding tension in your body and mind. On a more positive note, many postmenopausal women do not experience anxiety as a disorder but rather as a temporary, situational, emotional condition.

SITUATIONAL VERSUS GENERALIZED ANXIETY

Women express anxiety in various ways and to varying degrees. We will focus on the most common conditions: situational anxiety and generalized anxiety.

Situational anxiety typically is triggered by actual, external events. Examples include the risky behavior of an adolescent daughter, the progressive decline of a loved one with dementia, the big stretch that's required with taking on new job

DOI: 10.1201/9781003250968-9

responsibilities, or the anticipation about what to do in retirement. In contrast, *generalized anxiety* is a constant companion. It fluctuates in intensity and has no regard for events or situations. In fact, it is often out of proportion to existing events or situations. Some women seem to have a natural tendency toward anxiety in that their constitution is prone to worry. Feelings of apprehension and fear are especially prevalent, and ruminating thoughts tend to be mired in negativity.

During her care for women in the Breast Center at the University of Minnesota, Carolyn observed women of all ages waiting for results of their mammograms and ultrasounds. One 65-year-old woman brought to light the heightened situational anxiety that women can experience during these visits.

> *Kay's yearly screening mammograms had always had negative results. In fact, she had a negative exam just 5 months before our visit. Kay came in for an evaluation because she noted some tenderness and lumpiness in the outer area of her left breast. She was very worried because her best friend had been diagnosed recently with breast cancer and was undergoing chemotherapy. During Kay's breast exam, I did not detect a discrete mass but only some tenderness where the bra underwire pressed. I reassured Kay that this was likely benign, but we would look more closely at the area of concern with an ultrasound and a mammogram.*
>
> *As is typical for a busy breast center, Kay sat in the waiting room for over an hour while the radiologist evaluated her ultrasound and mammogram. When I came out to share the news that all was normal, Kay was frantically paging through a magazine and broke down crying as soon as she saw me. When she heard the good news, she hugged and thanked me profusely. Wiping away her tears, Kay revealed that while waiting for results, she had concluded she was dying and had made mental notes on planning her funeral and writing her obituary. She had even rehearsed how she was going to tell her family and friends this devastating news.*

Let's consider Kay's story from the perspective that anticipatory, situational anxiety could be beneficial. Kay's anticipation of the worst outcome may have been energizing. She used the waiting time to make plans and rehearse difficult conversations. Psychology suggests that, subconsciously, worrying can help you prepare for the worst: *"If I just worry enough about something happening, I'll be safe or it won't actually happen."* In this respect, Kay created a protective holding space while waiting for the news that could have had a profound impact on her life. Her joy at hearing the absence of cancer canceled the angst she felt in the waiting room.

Were Kay's ruminations extreme? Perhaps not, given that most women sitting in the waiting room are anticipating bad news. Yet, why exert so much energy worrying about what *might* happen? A better mental strategy might be for Kay to preserve her energy to deal with the known. In Kay's case, she could have worried far less.

We see worry as a strategy that your anxious brain can call on to deal with stress and uncertainty. Anxiety can help you navigate certain situations, or it can make situations even more nerve-wracking. We believe that you have a choice in how anxiety works for you at different times and in different situations.

When feelings of anxiety are extreme enough to interfere with your life, you may be dealing with a condition classified as a *generalized anxiety disorder*. The Anxiety and Depression Association of America estimates that 40 million people—almost one out of five people—suffer from an anxiety disorder, making it the most common mental health disorder in the United States.[1]

GENERALIZED ANXIETY DISORDER

Generalized anxiety disorder involves persistent and excessive worry that interferes with daily activities. This ongoing worry and tension may be accompanied by physical symptoms, such as restlessness, feeling on edge or easily fatigued, difficulty concentrating, muscle tension, or problems sleeping. Often, the worries focus on everyday things such as job responsibilities, personal health or the health of family members, financial matters, and other typical life circumstances.

Generalized anxiety is an epidemic in our society, with an estimated 25% of middle-aged women regularly taking an antidepressant.[2] Hormonal shifts account for some of this. The loss of estrogen and progesterone can heighten anxiety. Changes in the blood levels of estradiol and progesterone are associated with changes in mood regulation and cognition. Progesterone, in particular, is known to have calming and antianxiety benefits, but it is depleted after menopause, along with other hormones.

You may know women who struggle with feelings of hopelessness and negative self-talk, which trap them in a recurrent cycle. A single anxious thought can trigger intense physical symptoms. These can lead to avoidance behavior, which results in a cascade of negative thought patterns and feelings of isolation. This kind of pattern can overtake your thinking and prevent you from finding inner stillness in the present moment. In *The Power of Now*, Eckhart Tolle explains, "You are in the here and now, while your mind is in the future. This creates an 'anxiety gap,' where your mind is in a state of fear which prevents you from being present."[3]

June had experienced chronic anxiety for years. She came to her appointment, declaring that she was overcome with anxiety—she had reached her limit. She and her husband were now both retired and had been looking forward to enjoying long road trips together. However, June dreaded going on any kind of journey because of her considerable worry and fear that something bad would happen. On previous visits, I had encouraged June to consider an SSRI for anxiety, but she had declined. Now, I took additional time to explain that people with anxiety often focus on their fear of potential side effects and miss out on the benefits of medication. I told June that her anxious brain hates uncertainty and would rather suffer with what it knows, rather than risk trying something it doesn't know.

June was perplexed that in spite of her self-care efforts—including exercise, talk therapy, a meditation practice, and a recent visit with a massage therapist—she still felt anxious beyond reason. I made a frank appraisal, informing June that she had developed an anxiety disorder that could improve with medication. Because she was so desperate, June reluctantly agreed to try a low dose of an SSRI. She promised to take the medication for a 6-week trial—and to not read the package insert that would no doubt make her anxious about a multitude of potential side effects. On her return visit 6 weeks later, June appeared calm and collected. When I asked how she

was doing, without hesitation, she replied, "You changed my life. Despite my reluc-
tance, you insisted that I try medication, and your explanation of medication resis-
tance clicked for me. Admitting to myself that I had an anxiety disorder was the first
step, and realizing that a low dose of a medication could help me feel better was a
revelation. My irritability and ruminating thoughts are less, and I feel calmer and
better able to cope with day-to-day stressors. I am now able to see that my anxiety
was controlling me."

In June's case, her generalized anxiety had escalated into an actual disorder, and often, if untreated, anxiety can impair key functions of the brain such as memory, attention, and focus. While you may empathize with June's reluctance to take medication, when anxiety becomes pervasive and controlling, medication may be a necessary part of treatment. As June's anxiety lessened, she was able to manage her anxious feelings and feel more in control. At this stage in life, you may have reconciled that many things in life are not in your control. However, when it comes to coping with life stressors, there is comfort in realizing you have options for reducing responses that have a negative impact on your body and mind.

WHAT IS AN SSRI?

SSRIs, or selective serotonin reuptake inhibitors, are a type of antidepressant drug that increases the availability of serotonin in your nervous system. Serotonin carries signals between nerve cells and helps with many of your body's functions, including mood, sleep, and well-being. Commonly used SSRIs are citalopram (Celexa), fluoxetine (Prozac), and sertraline (Zoloft).

THE STRESS RESPONSE

Understanding more about your body's nervous system may give you some insight into your mindset and choice of strategies for dealing with stress. Feelings of anxiety, accompanied by worry and fear, keep your *sympathetic nervous system* activated. This is the part of the nervous system that signals your body's fight or flight response by triggering a mechanism called the hypothalamic-pituitary-adrenal axis (HPA). The hypothalamus alerts the pituitary gland (both in the brain) to release a hormone that will stimulate the adrenal glands (located just above your kidneys) to release the two main stress hormones: adrenaline and cortisol.

HYPOTHALAMIC-PITUITARY-ADRENAL AXIS

The HPA axis plays a critical role in your body's response to physical and psychological stressors. Dysregulations in the HPA axis have long been implicated in the development of depressive and anxiety symptoms.

Adrenaline and cortisol, which are released for a short period of time, rouse your body for emergency action. Your heart pounds, blood pressure rises, muscles tighten, breath quickens, and your senses become sharper. These are typical responses when your body is fighting off danger, facing a life-threatening or other traumatic event. However, many of us live is a state of chronic, low-level stress. Our lives are not being threatened, but we're short on time and have too much to do, often worrying about ourselves and everyone else. In this case, cortisol is released over a long period of time, and the result is detrimental. This cycle is called *stress hormone dysregulation*, and it causes an array of negative effects, making you feel stressed physically, emotionally, and mentally.

> *Arlena had been "over-the-top anxious" for most of her life. I knew her for many years because I had been her father's primary care physician. Both father and daughter were extremely talented and bright people; however, they had the same generalized anxiety disorder, and their frenetic personalities spread a wake of worry. I thought them both unquestionably candidates for medication to reduce their unrestrained, ruminating thoughts. Unfortunately, they were caught in an anxiety cycle, with the thought of taking medication so worrisome that it produced yet even more anxiety.*
>
> *I discussed with Arlena that her symptoms, including her worry and fear about taking medication, were clearly characteristic of generalized anxiety disorder. She would laugh and agree with the diagnosis but decline medication. Arlena was keenly aware of how her anxious state made work and home life difficult. Her compulsion to organize everyone's actions and movements drove colleagues and family members crazy. My suggestion to have Arlena set aside specific times to worry met with minimal success.*
>
> *It took over a year for Arlena to trust my advice and try a low dose of an SSRI to help moderate her anxiety. I didn't think that an SSRI alone would be enough to manage Arlena's highs and lows, and so I also encouraged her to start a meditation practice. Initially, she resisted saying, "I can't sit still with my crazy, intrusive thoughts for a moment. I can't calm my mind." However, although still skeptical, when she learned of a mindfulness-based stress response course that involved a walking meditation (rather than the typical sitting position), she decided to give it a try. The two interventions—medication and meditation—worked synergistically, and Arlena's anxiety level became more manageable.*

June and Arlena's stories illustrate differences between the anxious brain and the curious brain discussed in Chapter 2. When their anxious brains were activated, June and Arlena avoided trying medical treatment. However, when they engaged their curious brains, they saw that both medication and mindful approaches would ultimately be of benefit.

It's important to recognize that anxiety and curiosity are not simply the inverse of each other. A modest level of anxiety is necessary for alerting you to what's going on that needs your attention. This "good" kind of anxiety stimulates your curiosity to wonder about possibilities and to try something new or different.

BRIDGING THE GAP

We began this chapter by asking about your experiences with anxiety and its effect on your mental and physical health. As with the other postmenopausal conditions that we cover, adapting your lifestyle to manage various states of anxiety is important. You can navigate ordinary and extraordinary life experiences by using the integrative strategies we present below.

In conventional medicine, generalized anxiety disorder is usually treated with one of three groups of medications: SSRIs, SNRIs, and benzodiazepines. June and Arlena took medication that lessened their agitated and frenetic thoughts, minimizing their anxious state. However, these types of medications are not helpful for all women and are only partially beneficial for many. Practitioners often recommend a combination of medication and behavioral therapy. Cognitive-behavioral therapy with the right therapist can be a valuable resource for treating and rewiring your anxious brain.

COGNITIVE-BEHAVIORAL THERAPY

Cognitive-behavioral therapy is an evidence-based type of psychotherapy in which negative patterns of thought about the self and the world are challenged to alter unwanted behavior patterns or treat mood disorders. *Exposure therapy* reduces fear and anxiety by gradual exposure to the feared situation or object. *Somatic therapy* uses the mind-body connection to help you survey your internal self and listen to signals your body sends about areas of pain, discomfort, or imbalance. This allows you to learn more about the ways you hold on to your experiences in your body.

INTEGRATIVE STRATEGIES

Your feelings of anxiety can become stronger or weaker depending on how you respond to situations because your response affects the biological feedback to your nervous system. The primary neurotransmitters responsible for regulating levels of anxiety appear to be GABA and serotonin. You can practice integrative approaches to balance these neurotransmitters and to naturally feel better.

NEUROTRANSMITTERS

GABA (short for gamma-amino-butyric acid) is a neurotransmitter or chemical messenger, that allows communication between your brain and your nervous system. Its job is to modulate the balance between calming alpha brainwaves and energizing beta brainwaves. GABA has a calming effect on the brain and is your body's main inhibitory neurotransmitter. It may help to induce sleep and ease feelings of anxiousness.

Serotonin is a brain neurotransmitter derived from the amino acid tryptophan. It is key to regulating your appetite, mood, and melatonin production. The presence of serotonin in the brain is associated with a balanced emotional state, which is achieved in part by decreasing the activity of certain excitatory hormones, including dopamine and noradrenaline.

NOURISHMENT

A variety of practical tools and techniques are available to help you manage anxiety. We see these tools and techniques as nourishment for aligning your body and mind toward living a more peaceful and present-focused life. The World Health Organization's 2020 publication *Doing What Matters in Times of Stress: An Illustrated Guide* offers pragmatic tips and techniques for dealing with everyday stress.[4] For example, mindfulness and breath-based techniques are designed to reduce reactivity of the sympathetic nervous system to bring about a calmer, more relaxed state.

Be Present

Many inspirational authors have written about the need to quiet the mind and live more in the present moment. For example, the late Ram Dass (Richard Alpert) was an American Yogi well known for his teachings on spirituality, yoga, and medication. His 1971 book, *Be Here Now,* became the counterculture bible for thousands of young people seeking enlightenment during the darkness of the Vietnam War. It espoused the benefits of embarking on a spiritual journey to reach higher levels of consciousness through self-exploration.[5]

Another leading author on living a spiritual life is Pema Chodron, an American Buddhist monk. In *Taking the Leap, Freeing Ourselves from Old Habits and Fears,* Chodron asserts that Americans have lost tolerance for uncertainty.[6] She explains that we feel uneasy because every aspect of life is continually changing, yet we are always looking for a permanent fixed reference point that does not exist. Chodron recommends engaging in "micro-practices" to cope with the many uncertainties of daily living. Such practices can even help contend with phenomenal challenges, such as the COVID-19 pandemic.

You probably already use some type of micro-practice to connect with the present and calm your mind and spirit. One technique that can be done frequently throughout the day is to take a short pause, draw a deep breath, then let it go, and repeat two more times. Another approach is to identify places on your regular routes, such as murals, gardens, or tree-lined streets, that bring a smile or a feeling of gratitude. Spend some time in places that elicit a feeling of calm or joy, such as a park or green space or by a lake or river. Enjoy playful time with your pet—feel their joy. Anything that reminds you to pause and be present, away from constant worrying thoughts, will help quiet your mind. While these actions may seem too simple to have much effect, remember that small measures can create new habits and pathways. In the words of Eckhart Tolle, "unease, anxiety, tension, stress, worry—all forms of fear—are caused by too much future and not enough presence."[3]

Breath Work

When you appear anxious, someone often advises, *"Take a breath."* Although this might be irritating to hear, it is indeed beneficial to do. In *Breath*, James Neston identifies breath as the missing pillar of health and describes how harnessing the breath can support good health.[7] Neston tells an intriguing story of the hidden science behind conscious breathing practices that have been around for thousands of years. In a recurring cycle of loss and rediscovery, many of the techniques are being integrated into present-day knowledge for better health. Current research supports the benefits of various techniques such as diaphragmatic breathing, slow breathing, and alternate nostril breathing. Many approaches can be easily incorporated into your daily routine.

Two options to nurture relaxation are the 5.5 slow breath exercise and the 4–7–8 breathing exercise. *The 5.5 slow breath exercise* promotes autonomic changes that can increase relaxation, improve mood, spark new ideas, and reduce variability in heart rate.

1. Find a quiet spot, and sit or lie down comfortably. Relax your shoulders and belly.
2. Set a timer for 5 minutes.
3. Breathe in through your nose for 5 seconds. Expand your belly as air fills your lungs.
4. Without pausing, breathe out through your nose for 5 seconds. Bring the belly in as the lungs empty.
5. When the timer goes off, you're done.

The 4–7–8 breathing exercise is simple, takes almost no time, requires no equipment, and can be done anywhere. In this exercise, you always inhale quietly through your nose and exhale audibly through your mouth. Place the tip of your tongue against the ridge of tissue just behind your upper front teeth, and keep it there throughout the entire exercise. You will be exhaling through your mouth around your tongue; try pursing your lips slightly if this feels awkward. Exhaling takes twice as long as inhaling.

1. Exhale completely through your mouth, making a whoosh sound.
2. Close your mouth and inhale quietly through your nose for a count of *4*.
3. Hold your breath for a count of *7*.
4. Exhale completely through your mouth, making a whoosh sound for a count of *8*.
5. This is one breath. Now inhale again and repeat the cycle 3 more times.

If you have trouble holding your breath, speed up the exercise but keep to the ratio of 4:7:8 for the three cycles. With practice you can slow it down and get used to inhaling and exhaling more and more deeply.

Meditation and Mindfulness

Meditation has been practiced for many centuries in many cultures, each with its own language to describe the techniques and benefits. As a general term representing many approaches with common threads, meditation is essentially a state of being that involves the qualities of contemplation, introspection, nonjudgment, nonattachment, and higher awareness. In *Why Meditation Works*, James Baltzell, MD, explains meditation from a more conventional perspective. He divides meditation into three stages:[8]

- Physiological: the process of relaxing and achieving the relaxation response
- Insightful: gaining knowledge to your inner self and mind
- Spiritual: becoming aware of a higher consciousness

Meditation can be practiced with or without religious associations. One of the first challenges in learning to meditate is to find what school of meditation is right for you. Finding a class is often helpful, so start by looking in your community for options.

If you feel you can't meditate because your "mind is always racing" or you are "too hyper to sit still," try starting with this simple exercise:

- Sit comfortably.
- Focus on your breath, coming in and out.
- As soon as your mind gets distracted, simply redirect back to your breath.
- Start with 5 minutes, twice a day.

If a sitting meditation is difficult for you, then consider a walking meditation, or another meditation in motion using the experience of walking as the focus. A walking labyrinth is a pattern of pathways that weave in a concentric circle around a central point. You walk it slowly while quieting your mind. The process symbolizes the journey as much as the destination. Some women find meditative opportunities while gardening, driving along a clear stretch of road, or even while doing mindless domestic activities. As we've said, meditation is about quieting the mind in whatever ways work for you.

HeartMath is a way to help you learn to meditate (heartmath.com). This scientifically validated technique is a combination of hands-on and visual. It guides you to a state of relaxation intended to help manage stress, revitalize energy, and restore mental and emotional balance and resilience. When this technology is used, you can see a display of your heart rhythm, measured by heart rate variability, which indicates how your emotional state is affecting your nervous system. Having a visible measuring tool helps some women direct their breath to a calmer state. Heart rate variability can offer a window into the connection between your heart and your brain, which directly impacts how you feel and perform.

Mindfulness-Based Stress Reduction is the mindset of meditation. Mindfulness means being fully present in the here and now. It's about being aware, attentive, and immersed in each moment, and it can be done anytime and anywhere. Jon Kabat-Zinn, the leader in bringing the concept of mindfulness into both scientific and lay arenas, states, "Mindfulness means paying attention in a particular way: on purpose, in the present moment and nonjudgmentally."[9]

Mindfulness is one of the most effective and well-researched mind-body skills. More than 2,500 studies in the past 20 years have demonstrated the positive impact of mindfulness on physical, emotional, cognitive, and psychological well-being. Yet, most people completely underestimate its power. You might consider taking a class in mindfulness-based stress reduction, which can be a nonthreatening and easy way to begin exploring meditation. Classes are available in many areas of the country, both in-person and virtually.

Loving-Kindness Meditation stems back to the time of the Buddha more than 2,500 years ago. The Tibetan tradition, expressed in the mission of the Dalai Lama, has been influential in Western media's promotion of loving-kindness. It is about opening up the heart and cultivating love and compassion for ourselves and others. Doing so allows us to rise up and give what we most want to receive.

EXAMPLE OF A LOVING-KINDNESS MEDITATION

Breathe in through your nose slowly to the count of six, hold your breath for two counts, and exhale slowly to the count of six. Do this for a total of five breaths. With your hands resting on your lap or your heart, recite the loving-kindness phrases and try to generate feelings of kindness, friendliness, and compassion. Starting with yourself, say:

> *May I be free from fear. May I be free from suffering. May I be happy. May I be filled with loving-kindness.*

As you feel the warmth coming from your heart, imagine a dear friend or loved one and say:

> *May you be free from fear. May you be free from suffering. May you be happy. May you be filled with loving-kindness.*

Finally, extend the wish to all beings on the planet as you relax and say:

> *May all people everywhere be happy and filled with loving-kindness.*

Spend a few minutes allowing this wave of loving-kindness to swirl around and radiate from you.

Prayer

Prayer can be a variation on both meditation and mindfulness. Many women of post-menopausal age have been raised in a faith community and use prayer as a meditation or contemplative practice to enrich their connection with God or a higher power. Prayer can deepen one's faith and serve as a restorative and supportive practice. If prayer and a faith community give you sustenance, then use this as your discipline to stay centered when faced with anxious thoughts and worry.

Gratitude

Practicing and experiencing gratitude can help ease anxiety by allowing you to give a positive response of thanks and be in the present moment. Ralph Waldo Emerson advised that gratitude is a habit to be cultivated. We should recognize that every experience contributes to who we are; thus, we should express gratitude for all things.

We understand gratitude as a "state of thankfulness" or a "state of being grateful." It also involves a readiness to show appreciation for kindness and being able to return it. Gratitude is a state of both mind and body. It increases neural modulation in the brain, which regulates negative emotions. When gratitude is expressed, the brain releases dopamine and serotonin, two crucial neurotransmitters responsible for emotions that help you feel good. Gratitude is best practiced every day because it is all too easy to revert to an anxious mind. Practicing gratitude consistently will help strengthen your neural pathways so that, ultimately, being grateful becomes one of your enduring qualities. Brené Brown, an acclaimed research professor at the University of Houston, found that people who described themselves as joyful had one thing in common: an active gratitude practice. Other researchers have found that people who felt grateful and practiced gratitude journaling were happier and emotionally stronger than those who did not.

Sound Therapy

Have you ever tried using sound for healing or therapeutic purposes? Sara Auster, a sound therapist and author of *Sound Bath: Meditate, Heal and Connect Through Listening*, recommends instruments like singing bowls to initiate "a deeply immersive, full-body listening experience."[10] Singing bowls are metal bowls that can be tapped or rubbed with a wooden mallet to produce a vibrational bell-like sound and effect. Tibetan, or Himalayan, singing bowls were used for centuries by monks in Tibet and Nepal for spiritual and healing ceremonies. In recent years, the West has also discovered this technique as a promising treatment for stress. In fact, in one observational study, participants who experienced singing bowl sound meditation had significant reductions in tension, anxiety, depressed mood, and even physical pain scores.

Carolyn had an intense personal experience with sound therapy.

While at a retreat on integrative strategies for healing, I was struck by the power of sound bowls. One of the evening rituals was for us to gather in a room, lie on a mat, quiet our mind, and listen to the frequency and vibration of music that was being conducted by two music therapists. The sounds from the singing bowls and music surrounded me with a profound sense of well-being and clarity. I felt an immense peace and contentment that stayed with me for hours and was a perfect segue for a good night's sleep.

The exact mechanism for healing through singing bowl sounds is not known. One hypothesis is that brain waves may be significantly altered during sound healing, changing from a normal or even agitated state (such as beta waves) to an exceptionally relaxed state (such as theta or delta waves). Another theory is that the human body is surrounded by an energy field, which may interact with the vibrations of the instruments.

Forest Bathing

We can all relate to the beauty and healing nature of the outdoors, whether it be turquoise ocean waters, a snowcapped mountain range, or a birch tree forest. Forest therapy, also known as "Shinrin-Yoku" or Japanese forest bathing, is the practice of spending time in forested areas for the purpose of enhancing health, wellness, and happiness. In *The Outdoor Adventurer's Guide to Forest Bathing*, Suzanne Bartlett Hackenmiller, MD, describes ways of spending time in nature that invite healing interactions.[11] A framework for the practice requires the following elements:

- Your intention to connect with nature in a healing way
- Your patience to not rush through the experience

- Your focused and generous attention
- Your commitment to going beyond a one-time event
- Your mindset that the experience is not just about taking a walk but about deepening a relationship with nature by incorporating certain practices

Guides certified by the Association of Nature and Forest Therapy lead outdoor adventures and forest bathing experiences. Even without a guide, simply taking a mindful walk in a natural setting can do wonders for the soul. The power of the earth's resources to lighten your spirit and calm anxious thoughts is available to all of us.

Using the healing power of nature to transform health requires taking time to slow down and allow the essence of plants to take hold. Rudolf Steiner, the founder of Anthroposophic Medicine and Waldorf Schools, wrote extensively on the essence of plants and their energy and healing power. Plants have invisible elements of energy that are present for healing, yet are often overlooked in conventional medicine. Just as the most important interactions between people, such as love, are invisible, so too are the interactions in the plant kingdom. This is the value of forest bathing and why these experiences have become so sought after.

Emotional Freedom Technique

Also known as tapping, the emotional freedom technique (EFT) is a holistic healing process that can help resolve a range of issues, including stress, anxiety, phobias, and emotional disorders. If physical stimuli help you to calm your body, EFT can be beneficial.

Tapping therapy is based on the combined principles of ancient Chinese acupressure and modern energy psychology. It is used to restore the body to a balanced state. This simple tapping method uses two fingers on specific meridian endpoints of the body, depending on the condition to be treated. A major benefit is you can learn to do this on yourself. While progressing through the tapping sequence, you focus on the negative emotions or physical sensations you are experiencing and then reframe that emotion with a more positive message.

The method can be used with anyone dealing with anxiety and phobias, including women of all ages who either will not or cannot take medication for their anxiety. Carolyn recalls a patient who was highly vigilant about her health.

Angie ate the right foods, exercised regularly, and had a strong Christian faith and a supportive husband and friends. As a stay-at-home mother, four teenagers kept her on the run. Angie acknowledged that she tended to be on the "hyper side" but was not typically anxious. However, she began to experience episodes of racing heartbeat and tingling in her hands and feet, accompanied by a sense of impending doom. The intensity of her symptoms had sent her to the emergency room twice. From a conventional medicine perspective, she was clearly having panic attacks with an underlying generalized anxiety disorder.

Angie was feeling calmer when she saw me but still had racing thoughts and physical angst. She flatly refused my suggestion to take a very low dose of an SSRI. We then discussed using calming herbal products, taking magnesium at night, and listening to relaxation tapes. These strategies did not resolve her condition. Ultimately, Angie decided to consult an EFT practitioner to learn techniques to reduce her physical symptoms of panic. She found that the tapping techniques were helpful, especially when she felt a panic attack starting.

Supplements and Botanicals

So many products are on the market that promise relief from anxiety. The most useful supplements and herbs to help with an anxious state are those that support your body's natural balance of GABA and serotonin, the "feel good" neurotransmitters. Having a therapist by your side to help you evaluate how you respond psychologically to added supplements is often a wise decision.

5-HTP (5-hydroxytryptophan) is made naturally in the body and is commercially available as a product made from the seeds of a West African plant (*Griffonia simplicifolia*). Taking this supplement may boost serotonin levels because 5-HTP is converted from tryptophan into serotonin in the brain.

If you have anxiety but do not want to take an SSRI, a trial of 5-HPT might be beneficial. Start with a low dose of 50 mg at nighttime—but be forewarned that even a low dose might trigger more anxiety. If you are not having any side effects, you can incrementally increase the dose to 150 mg if needed. A word of caution is to avoid taking 5-HPT and an SSRI at the same time unless you are working with an integrative practitioner who is familiar with this combination.

I advise my patients to keep a simple diary of their symptoms, because it can be challenging to know whether any improvement in mood is from the supplement, situational, or possibly a placebo effect. An easy way to do this is to make a list of three or four symptoms that cause the greatest anxiety—eg, irritability, ruminating/negative thoughts, reactivity—and score them on a scale from 1 to 10. Then begin taking the supplement and repeat the scoring every week. Sometimes the benefit of a supplement is subtle, so keeping a diary of symptoms to identify any improvement is extremely helpful. Combining 5-HTP with a meditation practice has synergistic benefits, and anxiety lessens over time.

L-Theanine is an amino acid that has been studied for its use in promoting relaxation and calmness without causing drowsiness. This benefit seems to be related to the effect it has on the generation of alpha waves in the brain, which are believed to be associated with a relaxed yet alert mental status. It is also suggested that L-theanine increases GABA levels.

L-theanine is found in tea, which is a good way to naturally increase your intake. A cup of black tea (approximately 7 ounces) contains 18–30 mg of L-theanine and about 40 mg of caffeine, while a cup of green tea contains 6–12 mg of L-theanine and about 26 mg of caffeine. The ratio of L-theanine to caffeine is more desirable in green tea than in black tea, but green tea may still have more caffeine than you want. Therefore, supplementation with L-theanine may be a worthy option. Over-the-counter products typically have approximately 100 mg per capsule.

CBD has been gaining in popularity for many conditions, and early research is promising regarding its ability to help relieve anxiety. CBD can be derived from both hemp and marijuana plants. Hemp has been cultivated for many years and used to make clothing and various fiber products. However, because hemp and marijuana both come from cannabis plants, there is much confusion about the difference between the two compounds. So, what are the facts?

- The cannabis plant has several varieties, which contain different compounds called cannabinoids. CBD is a cannabinoid, as is tetrahydrocannabinol (THC).
- THC is a psychoactive compound—it is the stuff that gets you high.
- CBD products derived from hemp are a particular variety of the cannabis plant. They contain less than 0.3% THC and do not have any psychoactive effects. They are legal federally, but still illegal under some state laws.
- Marijuana is derived from varieties of the cannabis plant that contain much higher and varying amounts of THC. Marijuana is illegal federally, but legal under some state laws.

The biggest challenges regarding CBD products are standardization and knowing which variety to purchase. The FDA does not regulate CBD products, so it is up to you, the buyer, to choose quality products. Given the myriad laws and different state-to-state regulations affecting CBD products, the bottom line is to purchase trusted brands from reputable sources. To ensure the best quality extracts, check that the product has a certificate of analysis and that a reliable laboratory has conducted third-party testing. The highest-quality CBD companies adhere to what is known as current Good Manufacturing Practices (cGMP) to ensure you are getting the best CBD product on the market.

Food for Mood

If your belly is in a bad mood, so likely is your mind. What you eat can contribute to the development of mental health conditions, including depression and anxiety, as well as to their prevention and management. It is well known that unhealthy eating patterns can cause mood swings and blood sugar fluctuations. High-sugar foods, caffeine, and alcohol might flare anxiety. Food choices can interfere with the balance between the good bacteria (the anti-inflammatory bacteria) and the bad bacteria (the pro-inflammatory bacteria) in our gut. This is important because the bacteria in your gut also produce hundreds of neurochemicals that the brain uses to regulate basic psychological processes. For example, an estimated 90% of the body's serotonin—one of the "good" neurotransmitters that affect mood—is produced in the gut. Following a healthy whole food meal plan contributes significantly to a stable mood and can reduce flares of anxiety.

HEALING SYSTEMS

Homeopathy

Homeopathy is its own unique system of healing. Jacob Mirman, MD, author of *Demystifying Homeopathy* (originally published in 1994 as *What the Hell Is Homeopathy?*), describes homeopathy as an "energy medicine" that is backed by scientific evidence of almost 200 years.[12] It was a German physician, Dr. C. F. Samuel Hahnemann (1755–1843), who first codified principles into a system of medicine.

The guiding principle of homeopathy is *similia similibus curantur,* "let likes cure likes." This is markedly different from conventional medicine, which uses the law of opposites. For example, in conventional medicine, a patient with high blood pressure would be given medication to lower it. In homeopathy, the choice would be a substance that would induce high blood pressure because it is the energy of the substance that helps the body return to health. Another distinction of homeopathy is that the remedy is prepared through a series of dilutions, until there is no detectable chemical substance left in the solution. It is the energy of the substance, not the substance itself, that does the healing. As paradoxical as it seems, the more diluted the dose, the more potent the homeopathic remedy.

Homeopathic products are made from minerals, plants, animals, and other sources from the earth. The formulations are tiny pellets of various dilutions. Most homeopathic practitioners have extensive knowledge of materia medica from which they select a remedy.

MATERIA MEDICA

The *Materia Medica* is a book that lists the substances used in homeopathy along with detailed indications for their application. The information is compiled from provings and clinical observations.

My first experience with homeopathy was in the early 1980s when my mother came down with a severe case of shingles. Her left shoulder and arm had extensive blistering lesions which were extremely painful. In those days, no medication was available for shingles, so the patient had to wait out the natural course of the illness. Unfortunately, a common complication of shingles is post-herpetic neuralgia, a pain that persists well beyond the resolution of the lesions, and, in my mother's case, caused exacerbation of her anxiety. I happened to mention her condition to a colleague, Dr. Neil Nathan, a holistic physician with expertise in homeopathic medicine. He said that he had a remedy for pain and anxiety in the form of tiny pellets. My mother had never heard of homeopathy, yet within 24 hours of taking the remedy her pain subsided and her anxiety relieved. I don't know whether this result was the remedy, coincidence, or the placebo effect, but my mother was incredibly thankful.

Homeopathic medicine has two main categories of treatment: acute and chronic. Let's look at how they may be applied to anxiety.

Acute treatment is for illnesses that are self-limited and responsive to symptomatic relief. Homeopathic remedies can be used to treat different anxiety states and help you through an acute bout of anxiety or other minor illness. However, if the condition does not resolve, you need to ask for help.

Chronic treatment is typically needed for ongoing conditions, which require a comprehensive consultation with a trained homeopath practitioner who is skilled in obtaining a detailed history that reveals your physical, psychological, and emotional

Homeopathic Remedies for Acute Anxiety	
Remedy	**Use**
Aconitum napellus	Intense, sudden anxiety, panic, or fear
Argentum nitricum	Apprehension or stage fright associated with agitation
Arsenicum album	Deep anxiety about personal health
	Obsession with order and neatness

characteristics and concerns. For example, a chronic condition like generalized anxiety disorder is affected by many factors, including the nature of the problem, early health history, family medical history, previous treatment, and your inherent constitutional strength. The goal of the homeopath practitioner is to find the correct remedy that is most similar to your characteristics and symptoms. You can find a local practitioner by contacting the North American Society of Homeopaths.

EXERCISE

Exercise for the management of anxiety is a mainstay of integrative care. Adults who engage in regular physical activity experience fewer depressive and anxiety symptoms, thus supporting the notion that exercise offers a protective effect and/or is a self-management strategy to benefit mental health.

Studies from different disciplines also support this conclusion. Research in sports medicine has shown that regular aerobic exercise is associated with reduced activity of the sympathetic nervous system and hypothalamic-pituitary-adrenal axis. Psychologists studying how exercise relieves anxiety and depression suggest that a brisk 10-minute walk may be just as good for you as a 45-minute workout and can provide several hours of relief from anxiety. Numerous epidemiological studies have shown that exercise improves self-esteem and a sense of well-being. Exercise to mitigate anxiety is most effective when combined with other integrative strategies such as a meditation practice or cognitive-behavioral therapy.

Carolyn personally experiences how essential exercise is for her mental health.

If I didn't exercise, my anxiety would be unmanageable. Because this is so personal for me, I am continually telling women about the value of exercise and movement. When the word "exercise" elicits groans, I suggest choosing another concept like "movement" that doesn't sound so regimented. If a dance class, pickleball, or Zumba sounds more fun and less onerous than bike riding, running, or walking, then get engaged in that activity. I really don't care what you do, just so you do some movement.

We have discussed a variety of modalities that may quell your anxious state. No particular therapy is the answer: what works for you may not work for someone else. It's an individual journey to recognize in what ways, and to what extent, anxiety and accompanying thoughts may be controlling your actions or inactions. Do not let anxiety control your life. Anxiety is best approached from many perspectives, using a network of strategies. Reflect on the curious mind in Chapter 2. Experiment! Take the journey into wellness.

PATHWAYS TO CALM YOUR MIND

Self-Knowing: What is your story when it comes to experiencing anxiety? What are you already doing that helps settle your mind?

Self-Compassion: In what ways, if any, would you want to change your relationship with anxiety as you age?

Self-Advocacy: Are you interested in exploring any of the tools and techniques we have offered? If so, what would be your next step?

CATHERINE'S PATHWAY

When Carolyn insisted that we address anxiety as one of the common conditions of postmenopausal women, I must admit I felt this chapter was meant for others but not for me. I have known myself as calm and grounded with a resilient core. Sure, I had occasional bouts with anxiety—what mother of a rebellious teen doesn't—but these were temporary, or what Carolyn and I term, "situational." But I learned while working on this chapter that although "generalized anxiety" doesn't fit my profile, I have had stretches of anxiety over different situations: my daughter's risky behaviors, divorce (twice), illnesses and deaths of family and friends, my own breast cancer, and professional challenges. Decades ago, a colleague and friend likened me to a swan, gliding along on the surface but paddling like mad underneath. It's an apt description of someone who seeks a life of connection and harmony and must find ways to counteract negative feelings.

In that spirit, I have engaged in a variety of healing modalities, adapted my lifestyle to include more exercise and better nutrition, and broadened my perspectives through immersive experiences in other cultures and countries. Essential constants for me are being with family and friends and, since 2007, working out with my personal trainer on a weekly basis.

About 15 years ago, while experiencing an especially rough patch in my personal life, I sought help from both a psychotherapist and a hypnotherapist, both of whom helped me regain my equilibrium. While working on this book, I was faced with a cluster of major life stresses. I found that exercise, nutrition, sleep, and saying "no" weren't quite sufficient to ease my anxieties. So, I sought further help in the form of antianxiety medication. There, I claim it: anxiety. I don't know how long I will be taking this medication, but it is a welcome assist to my own self-care.

I had planned to experience forest bathing sometime in the future and then the experience presented itself in late 2021 when I visited my friend Gretchen at her home in Accompong, Jamaica. In this mountainous region of lush vegetation (trees of palm, banana, coconut, poinsettia), soothing moisture, and cooling breezes, I found the perfect antidote to anxiety. I felt the benevolent spirits as we sat near the sacred Kindrah tree—symbolizing One Family—where in 1739, four warring tribes united to maintain their independence from the British. The Maroon culture, so alive with tradition, is about living in the present and being with nature. For me, the culture, environment, and friendships are ideal for knowing harmony.

8 Fatigue
Enhance Resilience

"I don't feel like myself" is a common refrain, along with, "I just don't feel well. I feel so tired. I want more energy." There isn't a medical diagnostic code for "not feeling myself," yet many postmenopausal women do feel a loss of vitality and energy. This is not the fatigue associated with cancer treatment or other chronic diseases. Rather, it is the run-of-the-mill, generally not feeling good, lack of energy, "no pep" type of fatigue. Loss of vitality does not have to coincide with aging. There are solutions to restoring your energy and optimizing your overall health.

Fatigue Is Multifactorial

Fatigue may be physical or mental, or both. The experience of fatigue likely differs from person to person. You may describe your fatigue as feeling run-down, tired, exhausted, listless, melancholy, unmotivated, or simply having low energy. Your brain might feel like it's running on empty and in need of a recharge.

> *Amy, age 60, came to me for an integrative consult with a main concern of fatigue. She reported that her life was good: her marriage was stable, her children were grown and healthy, and her financial situation was comfortable. She also had begun seeing a naturopath who was very encouraging and supportive in improving Amy's health and well-being. Amy was also completing a health coach program to guide women through health crises. However, she appeared to be in the midst of her own health crisis. For our consult, she brought a lengthy list of concerns that included not feeling well, poor energy, midday fatigue, belching, bloating, stomach pain, constipation, weight gain, muscle aches, body pain, hair thinning, anxiety, depression, and insomnia. Her symptoms had escalated over the previous 5 years, during which time she had seen many physicians. She had been prescribed lots of medications and supplements and carried multiple diagnoses: fibromyalgia, chronic fatigue, generalized anxiety disorder, gastroesophageal reflux disease, irritable bowel syndrome, osteoporosis, hyperlipidemia, and chronic insomnia. Every body system was dysfunctional. Amy was out of balance.*

Lest you think Amy's story is atypical—could anyone really have all these things wrong with her and still be functioning?—the truth is that many women do have multiple system dysfunction and are simply managing day by day. These are the tales of dysregulation, often generalized by practitioners as "fatigue." Women who say they have fatigue and related symptoms have often been told that the results of their exam and lab tests are all normal, so the problem must be psychological. We know that at times fatigue can be related to mood disorders, but often it is a physiological dysfunction that needs to be addressed.

DOI: 10.1201/9781003250968-10

BRIDGING THE GAP

Health practitioners usually dread hearing "fatigue" as the reason for an appointment because often there is no clear test to diagnose the problem and no easy solution. Fatigue tends to get directed into the realm of mental health, and depression becomes the focus of treatment. However, many women with fatigue are not depressed and do not accept the diagnosis or the label. Women feel frustrated when their healthcare providers do not acknowledge the impact that fatigue has on their quality of life. They feel dismissed when an underlying pathology is not identified or a fitting solution is not investigated. While an easy fix may be hard to find, effective options, fortunately, are available to mitigate fatigue from an integrative perspective.

INTEGRATIVE STRATEGIES

For some women who suffer from "not feeling well" early in their postmenopausal years, estrogen therapy may help to resolve symptoms of fatigue and low energy. In such cases, supporting the hormonal state helps restore overall balance. Sometimes, tweaking a thyroid condition with natural thyroid replacement hormone or restoring sleep can reestablish vitality. However, most of the time, treatment for fatigue is a complex condition with many layers to peel back before energy and better health can be restored. The strategies for better health may require subtle changes or substantial lifestyle shifts to restore and rebalance the whole-body state. A holistic practitioner may often be needed to facilitate the deeper aspects of health needed to heal.

Understanding some of the trending terminology associated with causes of fatigue and rehabilitation of energy might be helpful.

Detoxification is the body's way of getting rid of toxins that could otherwise build up and interfere with health. The liver is the main site of whole-body detox, through various pathways that eliminate and neutralize toxins. Our bodies were designed to handle stress, detoxify chemicals, and preserve cell function, but when the burden increases, those naturally built-in systems can't keep up with demand. Signs of poor detox include fatigue, difficulty concentrating, and unexplained aches and pains. Detoxification can be optimized by making diet and lifestyle changes to support good cellular cleaning processes.

Oxidative stress is what happens when our cells are attacked by free radicals, which are unstable molecules that damage the body. During our lifetime, we are exposed to many external toxins (eg, smoking, alcohol, poor diet, chronic stress, pollution) that can damage our cells. Healthy cells can make enzymes to counteract oxidative damage, but unhealthy cells cannot. If oxidative stress is not managed, it can contribute to chronic inflammation and a state of fatigue. The use of antioxidants can neutralize free radicals before they cause too much damage. For example, consuming a good diet and maintaining a healthy lifestyle can help lower oxidative burden and result in better health.

Methylation is a biochemical process of DNA repair that makes sure every cell is functioning optimally. When specific compounds attach to a molecule, it acts like a "green light." This process allows the molecule to do its work and regulate the activities of the body. When methylation is going well, your cardiovascular, neurological, reproductive, and detoxification system are optimized. When it is not going well, fatigue is the most common symptom. A genetic variant in an enzyme named MTHFR can contribute to poor methylation. You can improve the methylation cycle by eating healthy, whole-foods and essential B vitamins.

Stress response can't be ignored when considering the impact that stress has on fatigue. We talk about the stress response in Chapter 7, and to summarize, stress will activate the sympathetic nervous system, which in turn activates the adrenal glands to release the stress hormone, cortisol. With cortisol circulating throughout the day, the body is in a chronic low-level stress response that keeps the body revved up and on high alert. This alert state can eventually lead to exhaustion and fatigue.

These processes need to be optimized as they influence every aspect of your physiology and, subsequently, your physical and mental health.

Nourishment

Digestive Health

Many women who lack energy or vitality often carry a lifelong history of irritable bowel syndrome, a condition that can include symptoms of bloating, gas, belching, abdominal pain, constipation, and loose stools or diarrhea. Maybe your digestion has not been good for years, and you have been on and off a variety of drugs and digestive products, including antacids, proton-pump inhibitors, stool softeners, or laxatives, to manage your symptoms. Central to an integrative approach is restoring health by improving digestion through nourishing foods. Healing the gut reduces systemic inflammation, improves nutrient absorption, enhances immune responses, and supports an optimal microbiome.

GASTROINTESTINAL CONDITIONS

Irritable bowel syndrome (IBS) is a common gastrointestinal disorder affecting 7%–21% of the general population. Symptoms can include cramping, abdominal pain, bloating, diarrhea, and constipation.

IBS-C: the abdominal discomfort or bloating happens with constipation (stools passing less than three times per week). The stool is often hard and difficult to pass. There may be a feeling of incomplete emptying.

IBS-D: the abdominal discomfort or bloating happens along with stools that are often loose and watery. Stools may be passed multiple times during the day.

Small intestinal bacterial overgrowth occurs when bacteria that normally grow in other parts of the gut start growing in the small intestine. The result is pain and diarrhea. It can also lead to malnutrition as the bacteria start to use up the body's nutrients.

Not that long ago, conventional gastroenterologists gave little credit to the gut for being more than a drainage system for waste. Recently, however, attention has been given to the essential value of the gastrointestinal (GI) system and its microbiome. The gut is an important interface with our environment, with a surface area of about 450 square feet larger than that of our skin. Let's look more closely at the essential components of the GI tract and how proper functioning of your digestive system can reboot your energy and overall well-being.

Understanding Your Gut

The GI tract, from mouth to anus, is one of the most complex systems in the body. It is often called the "second brain." It functions in concert with the immune, endocrine, and nervous systems, which is why having a healthy gut is a foundation for good health. The GI tract is home to the enteric nervous system, the gut-associated lymphatic tissue (GALT), the microbiome, and the gut lining. Each plays a vital role in GI health and the gut-brain connection. Let's look at each component separately.

The *enteric nervous system* is a subdivision of the peripheral nervous system; it is composed of millions of nerve cells that line the entire GI tract, and its function is to directly control the GI system. This gut-brain connection continuously sends biochemical signals between the enteric nervous system and the central nervous system via the vagus nerve. It is the work of the vagus nerve when you have a "gut feeling" or feel butterflies in your stomach.

THE VAGUS NERVE

The vagus nerve is the longest nerve of the autonomic nervous system. It transmits messages about heart rate, blood pressure, stress response, and digestion. It connects the "rest and digest" part of the nervous system and can make you feel calm.

Gut-associated lymphoid tissue is the largest mass of lymphoid tissue in the body and is situated throughout the GI tract. It consists of many types of immune cells, including lymphocytes, as well as collections of tissues involved in immune function, such as the tonsils. The role of GALT is to manage your immune response from the massive antigen exposure experienced by the gut and help prevent you from getting an infection. It's your gut that fights off environmental and food toxins that enter your body. GALT depends on a healthy intestinal microbiome to function at its best.

Microbiome refers to the trillions of bacteria, viruses, and fungi that normally live inside all of us, mostly in the large intestine. These microscopic organisms help perform important tasks in the body. They digest food to generate nutrients for our cells, synthesize vitamins, metabolize drugs, detoxify carcinogens, stimulate renewal of cells in the gut lining, and activate and support the immune system. Keeping this diverse environment healthy is essential to maintaining good gut health. However, this environment is continuously exposed to various stress factors associated with modern lifestyles, as well as food additives and contaminants such as heavy metals, pesticides, antibiotics, organic pollutants, and other toxins. Over time, this can result in the microorganisms becoming unhealthy and getting out of balance, causing dysbiosis.

DYSBIOSIS

Dysbiosis is a term for an "imbalance" in the microbial environment of the GI tract. It is associated with intestinal disorders including inflammatory bowel disease, irritable bowel syndrome, and a number of disorders outside the GI tract, such as allergy, asthma, metabolic syndrome, cardiovascular disease, and obesity.

The foods you eat directly influence your gut microbiome. For example, a diet high in fiber fuels the gut bacteria, helps maintain the gut wall, modulates blood sugar, and manufactures essential molecules that benefit your well-being. Another example is the production of neurotransmitters: 90% of the body's serotonin is made in the digestive tract. This neurotransmitter is essential for mood and brain support, again demonstrating the importance of the gut-brain connection. When the microbiome is unbalanced and not functioning optimally, you might experience mood changes, fatigue, headaches, and sleep issues, not just GI symptoms.

Gut lining is the extensive intestinal lining, inside your GI tract, that covers more than 4,000 square feet of surface area. When the gut lining is working properly, it forms a barrier that prevents most large molecules and germs from being absorbed into the bloodstream. When the gut lining is not working properly, small gaps in the barrier allow unwelcome bacteria and food particles to cross. This harmful condition is called intestinal permeability or leaky gut.

Leaky guts allow food particles and bacteria to spill into the bloodstream, causing symptoms such as fatigue, weight gain, digestive discomfort, achy joints, and even skin problems. When food particles escape from the intestinal tract, your body

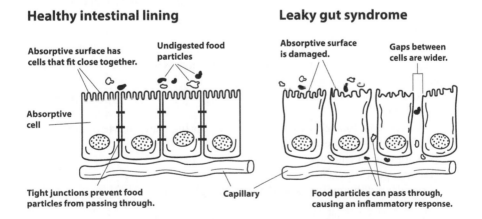

now recognizes them as foreign substances. Your immune system goes into attack mode and produces antibodies, which can trigger food allergies and also result in inflammation. As this continues, it's easy to see that individuals with a leaky gut may develop chronic health conditions.

Healing Your Gut: An Elimination Diet

If you suffer from low energy, fatigue, and poor gut health, you may want to try an elimination diet or a rejuvenation eating plan. Some women are curious about this path and want to explore it, while others reject it out of hand. Being open with how you feel about it will allow your practitioner to determine how to implement or modify an elimination diet for you, or whether to even advise trying it.

An elimination diet has multiple purposes: to identify hidden food allergens, to improve your body's ability to detoxify and excrete substances that may be causing symptoms, and to support the function of your immune system. Every day, you are exposed to toxins in the environment, such as chemicals, pesticides, medications, food-borne toxins, and alcohol. Unhealthy gut bacteria sometimes also make toxins. As these toxins accumulate in your body over time, the demand on your liver to detoxify them becomes greater. If your diet doesn't provide enough of the appropriate nutrients or your digestive system is not working properly, the liver can become overwhelmed. The result? Symptoms of chronic ill-health, including fatigue.

Everyone's biochemistry is unique, so a tailored approach is needed. An elimination diet calls for commitment and willingness to change—the kind of change that will quickly translate into improved function, vitality, and energy. We favor the diet plan detailed in Jeffrey Bland's *The 20-Day Rejuvenation Diet Program*.[1] His guide articulates fundamental principles and provides a methodical plan for healthy eating. Another reference for an elimination diet is *The Wahls Protocol*.[2] Dr. Terri Wahls advises 100 days of an elimination diet that aggressively intervenes against inflammation by reducing foods that tend to promote it. Many other contemporary books spell out elimination diet plans that may also be beneficial.

Here are some general guidelines that are part of most elimination diet plans:

- Eat a wide variety of foods, including rice, oatmeal, beans, vegetables and fruits (except citrus), nuts and seeds, olive oil, ghee, chicken, turkey, lamb, and fish.
- Avoid dairy products, wheat (gluten), corn, eggs, coffee, alcohol, refined sugars, trans fats, corn oil, food additives/preservatives, or processed foods.
- Avoid any foods to which you have a known sensitivity. Soy and citrus are common.
- Drink at least four glasses of water a day. Spring water and herbal teas are preferred to other beverages.
- Do not restrict calories.
- Eat at regular times of the day.
- Consider a daily multivitamin/mineral supplement.

The first few days of the program may be challenging to follow. You may even feel worse initially, but most women feel remarkably healthier in a week's time, reporting they feel "energized and clear-headed." This experience may offer you a glimpse into feeling better—and may even be the first time in years that life seems hopeful.

After the first phase of the elimination diet plan, foods can then be reintroduced, but this must be done methodically—adding one food at a time and paying careful attention to how your body responds both physically and emotionally. We strongly encourage you to work with a practitioner trained in integrative medicine or functional medicine who can guide you on the path to success.

Testing the Gut

If an elimination diet is not realistic for you or if you have not had success with one, testing for food allergies or nutritional deficiencies may be helpful. Many labs offer comprehensive testing of blood and urine to evaluate well over a hundred biomarkers that assess your body's functional need for antioxidants, vitamins, minerals, essential fatty acids, amino acids, digestive support, and other select nutrients. Personalized recommendations are also often provided based on the results. Digestive health can also be assessed through a comprehensive stool profile—a group of advanced stool tests that provide clinical information that can be used to manage gastrointestinal health. These tests are not typically ordered by conventional medicine practitioners, so consulting with an integrative-holistic practitioner is often necessary.

Provoking the Gut

Many triggering foods can make your gut unhealthy. Conversely, many foods can support a healthy gut and microbiome. Making dietary changes is often essential to restore your gut health and improve your energy level.

Before we talk about a few specific recommendations, what's the story on gluten? *Gluten* is a general term for the proteins found in wheat, rye, barley, triticale, and many other types of foods. It is theorized that breakdown products of gluten bind to cells of the gut lining, signaling them to secrete too much of a protein called zonulin. Secreted zonulin binds to the cells of the gut lining, which ultimately results in small gaps in the barrier of the gut wall. When this happens, you can develop intestinal permeability or leaky gut, which was discussed earlier in this chapter.

Some people have an immune reaction to eating gluten, a condition that is called celiac disease. If you have celiac disease, you will need to completely remove all gluten products from your diet. Fortunately, celiac disease is not very common, affecting only about 1% of the people in the United States. However, if you have tested negative for celiac disease but still have lots of digestive issues, it is possible you have what is called *gluten intolerance*, also known as *non-celiac gluten sensitivity*. A larger percentage of people, 6% or more, have gluten intolerance, and another 1% have a non-celiac wheat sensitivity. If you have gluten intolerance, removing gluten from your diet resolves symptoms, even though you have tested negative for celiac disease.

CELIAC DISEASE

Celiac disease is an autoimmune disease seen in genetically predisposed people in whom ingesting gluten leads to damage of the small intestine. Over time, the damaged small intestine can result in malabsorption of nutrients and, eventually, malnutrition. Gluten is found in wheat, rye, barley, and other food products. Celiac disease can manifest through gastrointestinal symptoms such as stomach cramps, bloating, gas, vomiting, and diarrhea. Long term, these can lead to weight loss, failure to thrive, and delayed growth and puberty.

Gluten intolerance causes symptoms similar to those of celiac disease, although individuals with gluten intolerance do not test positive for celiac disease and symptoms resolve when gluten is removed from the diet.

Wheat allergy is different from both celiac disease and gluten intolerance. In this condition, the immune system overreacts to one of the proteins found in wheat, resulting in hay fever, wheezing, rash (eczema/hives), gastrointestinal upset, and other symptoms.

Once you have determined whether gluten or wheat is causing a problem for you (and addressed it if needed), a few recommendations are typically helpful across the board. These include avoiding simple sugars, minimizing alcohol, and eating a diet low in fermentable carbohydrates.

Simple sugars are a form of carbohydrate. They are digested by enzymes in the small intestine and rapidly absorbed into the bloodstream. The two most common simple sugars are glucose and fructose, which together make up sucrose or common sugar. Approximately 48% of the caloric intake in the American diet is carbohydrates, with 13% coming from added sugars. The excess sugar in our diet has contributed to numerous diseases, including metabolic syndrome, obesity, diabetes, cardiovascular disease, liver disease, tooth decay, and even cognitive conditions. While ingesting more simple sugars and less dietary fiber is believed to have lasting and detrimental effects on your microbiome, the exact mechanism is not yet fully understood. What we do know is that decreasing your intake of simple sugars and increasing your intake of healthier complex carbohydrates that take longer to be digested will benefit your gut microbiome.

Fructose is another simple sugar that is primarily either combined with glucose (to form sucrose) or is a component of high-fructose corn syrup, which is added as a sweetener to processed foods and carbonated beverages. Start reading labels, and you will be shocked to see how many food products contain added sucrose and high-fructose corn syrup. Increased consumption of fructose is a major contributor to nonalcoholic fatty liver disease, high cholesterol, insulin resistance, and diabetes. Emerging studies also show that fructose metabolism in the liver and intestine contributes to changes in the gut microbiome.

Alcohol intake should be limited for many reasons. First, women are less tolerant of alcohol than men, and this intolerance increases after menopause. The enzyme that metabolizes alcohol in the liver—alcohol dehydrogenase—becomes less efficient as we age. Second, your body loses water volume as you age. This means that you are more easily dehydrated and that any form of alcohol in your body is not easily diluted. Third, alcohol is a depressant that has many downstream effects on the body. It exacerbates poor-quality sleep, which leads to increased fatigue, decreased alertness, and impaired cognitive performance. Fourth, alcohol also affects the microbiome and, along with an increased intestinal permeability, can create digestive issues.

But we understand—and like an occasional glass of wine, too! Our best advice is to set your limit at two drinks a week. The common belief that a glass of wine in the evening is a health benefit may not be advisable, especially if you suffer from fatigue.

Fermentable carbohydrates often go by the acronym FODMAPS, which stands for fermentable oligo-, di-, monosaccharides, and polyols. In sensitive people, this group of carbohydrates can aggravate gut symptoms such as bloating, gas, and stomach pain. A diet low in FODMAPS is recommended for the management of irritable bowel syndrome. A diet low in FODMAPS restricts these high-FODMAP foods:

- Oligosaccharides: wheat, rye, legumes, garlic, onions
- Disaccharides: milk, yogurt, soft cheese (main carb is lactose)
- Monosaccharides: various fruits, including apples, apricots, cherries, figs, mangoes, nectarines, peaches, pears, and plums; sweeteners such as honey and agave nectar (main carb is fructose)
- Polyols: certain fruits and vegetables, including blackberries and lychee; mannitol and sorbitol, which is found in some sugar-free gum

Supporting the Gut

Whole-Foods Plant-Based (WFPB) Diet: The WFPB diet is more of a lifestyle than a set diet. The basic principle of a WFPB diet is to focus on plants. Vegetables, fruits, whole grains, legumes, beans, seeds, and nuts should make up the majority of what you eat.

WHOLE FOODS

Whole foods are foods that remain close to their state in nature. They do not have added sugars, starches, flavorings, or other manufactured ingredients. They are the opposite of foods that are processed in a factory.

Many proponents of the WFPB diet promote locally sourced, organic food whenever possible. WFPB diets include the following foods:

- Foods dense in nutrients, including leafy greens, collard greens, and kale
- Fruits with a low glycemic index, such as berries, cherries, and plums
- Healthy fats, such as avocados, olive oil, grass-fed butter, and ghee
- Clean protein, such as organic grass-fed beef, pasture-raised poultry, lamb, wild-caught fish, wild game, and free-range eggs
- Herbs and spices

Fiber is a special type of carbohydrate. The importance of fiber for digestion and general health as we age cannot be stressed enough. Adequate intake of dietary fiber is increasingly recommended as a means to maintain and increase health and well-being and improve the gut microbiome. You need at least 20–30 grams of fiber per day for good health, but most Americans get only about 15 grams per day. Great sources of fiber are whole fruits and vegetables, whole grains, and beans.

You can easily figure the approximate amount of fiber you're getting in your diet. Write down everything you eat in a typical 24-hour period and then search online for the number of grams of fiber in each food. For example, enter "grams of fiber in an avocado" into Google or your favorite search engine. Add up all the grams of fiber to estimate your daily intake.

DIETARY FIBER

Dietary fiber is the part of plant-based food that passes through the digestive system mostly without breaking down or being digested. There are two types of fiber: soluble and insoluble. Most plants contain both types but in different amounts.

Soluble fiber dissolves in water and can help lower blood levels of glucose and cholesterol. Foods with soluble fiber include oatmeal, nuts, beans, lentils, apples, and blueberries. Soluble fiber includes plant pectin and gums, including psyllium.

Insoluble fiber doesn't dissolve in water and can help food move through the digestive system, promoting regularity and preventing constipation. Foods with insoluble fiber include wheat bread, couscous, brown rice, legumes, carrots, cucumbers, and tomatoes.

Functional fibers (prebiotics) are isolated nondigestible carbohydrates that resist digestion in the small intestine and reach the colon, where they are fermented by the gut microflora and stimulate the growth of intestinal bacteria. Prebiotics are found naturally in foods such as leeks, asparagus, chicory, Jerusalem artichokes, garlic, onions, wheat, oats, and soybeans.

Digestive enzymes can help restore the level of stomach acid, which decreases as we age. Some individuals require enzymes in supplemental form (eg, protease, bromelain, amylase, and lipase) to assist in proper food digestion and absorption. Enzymes are often depleted in foods that have been overcooked or overprocessed. In addition, when we multitask and eat while doing other activities, our bodies are not clued into the need to secrete the necessary enzymes for digestion.

You may find that taking one or two capsules of digestive enzymes 30 minutes before eating or with your meal helps with digestive issues. Also, there are natural digestive enzymes that aid in digestion such as pineapples, papayas, mangoes, and honey, as well as fermented foods like kefir, sauerkraut, and kimchi. In Ayurvedic medicine, it is not uncommon to begin the meal with a small glass of bitters to help your stomach release more gastric juices and prepare for digestion.

Prebiotics are specialized plant fibers that are not digestible but can exert beneficial effects by stimulating growth or activity of microorganisms that are present in the intestine. Not all fibers are prebiotic, but all prebiotics can be classed as fiber. Some prebiotics are found naturally in foods such as leeks, asparagus, chicory, Jerusalem artichokes, garlic, onions, wheat, oats, and soybeans. Other foodstuffs have been fortified with prebiotic ingredients such as inulin and oligofructose. The value of prebiotic substances is that they are available as substrates for probiotics.

Probiotics are live microorganisms that help balance your microbiome and keep your digestive system functioning properly. Clinical trials suggest that exposure to healthy microbes through the gastrointestinal tract powerfully shapes immune function. Multiple studies have indicated that probiotics containing a blend of lactobacilli, bifidobacteria, and streptococci can provide optimal support for a diverse range of health needs. Think of probiotics as the beneficial microorganisms that help fight the microscopic harmful bugs that cause inflammation and other problems in your gut.

Probiotics can be found in foods such as yogurt, cheese, miso, sauerkraut, and kimchi. They are also available as a supplement form. When selecting a probiotic, look for products that contain these five core bacteria:

- *Lactobacillus plantarum*
- *Lactobacillus acidophilus*
- *Lactobacillus brevis*
- *Bifidobacterium lactis*
- *Bifidobacterium longum*

Integrative medicine has been a proponent of probiotics for years, yet active debate continues about their benefits. Conventional medicine does not endorse their use and awaits evidence-based guidelines and conclusive research before recommending supplementation. However, conducting research is challenging because different probiotics contain different strains of bacteria (with varying benefits), and many probiotic products contain more than one strain.

When purchasing probiotic supplements, buy from a trusted retailer and look for a seal from a third-party certifier. Reputable supplements should list the genus, species, and strain of bacteria. Also check the label for the number of organisms (listed as colony-forming units, or CFU) that will be alive by the use-by date and the dose. Doses for adults typically range from 1 billion to 40 billion CFUs—a wide range, which makes selecting a product difficult for the consumer. You can choose from an array of tablets, powders, and liquids, depending on the form you prefer.

A *fecal microbiota transplant* (FMT) is exactly what it sounds like—collecting fecal material from a healthy person and transplanting it into an ill person. FMT can increase the microbial diversity of the intestines, maintain the microbial balance within the intestines, and rebuild the function of the immune system. The first Microbiota Therapeutics Program was started at the University of Minnesota in 2012 by Dr. Alexander Khoruts. This microbiota donor program recruits healthy individuals to donate stool samples that can be turned into microbial transplants in the form of capsules that are taken orally. This is currently used to treat individuals with *Clostridioides difficile* (often called just *C diff*), a bacterial infection of the gut. In this rapidly growing area, it appears that FMT may be helpful in other conditions like inflammatory bowel disease.

Immune Support

We know that the immune system gets weaker as we age, thus postmenopausal women need to consider factors that will help slow down the immunological clock. In his 2020 revision of *From Fatigued to Fantastic*, Dr. Jacob Teitelbaum suggests multiple ways to support the immune system, including naming beneficial supplements and botanicals that can reduce fatigue and improve overall health.[3]

The COVID-19 pandemic is a dramatic illustration of an environmental challenge to your immune system because it forces you to stay indoors more than usual or desirable and adds high stress levels that can affect your mental and physical health. Holistic practices, including quality sleep, good nutrition, physical activity, social support, and stress management, can foster a strong baseline of health. Dr. Teitelbaum and many integrative practitioners recommend the following basic supplements:

- Vitamin C 500 mg twice a day
- Vitamin B complex (contains eight B vitamins)
- Quercetin 250 mg per day
- Melatonin beginning with 0.3 mg and increasing as tolerated to 2 mg at night to improve sleep
- Vitamin D_3 1,000–3,000 IUs per day
- Zinc 30–50 mg per day

Antioxidants

Antioxidants are substances that reduce oxidative stress and protect our bodies from the damaging effects of free radicals. The following are particularly beneficial for fatigue.

Alpha lipoic acid is a nutritional coenzyme that is involved in the metabolism of proteins, carbohydrates, and fats for energy production. It is also necessary to transport glucose from the bloodstream into our body's cells. In addition, lipoic acid is called the universal antioxidant because it can scavenge a number of free radicals. The cells and tissues in your body are continually threatened by damage caused by toxins from free radicals, reactive oxygen species (which are produced during normal oxygen metabolism), and from the environment. Free radicals, once formed, can disrupt metabolic function and cell structure. Alpha lipoic acid is often added to a mixture of supplements when restoring the body after an illness or when struggling to restore energy. A dose of 100–300 mg per day is typical, but it is best to seek advice from a trained functional medicine practitioner.

Coenzyme Q_{10} (CoQ_{10}) is naturally found in every cell in the body. Although its primary role involves energy production, it acts as an antioxidant, which protects cells from damage and plays an important part in metabolism. Although CoQ_{10} is found in foods like meat, fish, and nuts, the amount in these dietary sources isn't enough to significantly increase your CoQ_{10} levels.

CoQ_{10} levels are lower in people with certain conditions, such as heart disease and chronic fatigue syndrome, and in those who take statins, which are drugs that lower cholesterol. CoQ_{10} levels also decrease as we age, so taking a supplement as you grow older can help support optimal energy levels. The most commonly available products are ubiquinol and ubiquinone. Both are valid forms of CoQ_{10}, but ubiquinol is better absorbed. A typical dose of 100 mg is considered safe and is available in capsule, chewable tablet, and liquid form.

Folate is an essential vitamin (B_9) that works together with the other B vitamins and plays a vital role in methylation. Folate also helps maintain brain, nerve, and blood cells, and it contributes to DNA health. Folate is found in numerous foods, including leafy greens, legumes, and asparagus. The synthetic form is called folic acid, commonly used in supplements and fortified foods, but it is less beneficial than natural folate. Genetic variation affects the availability and the requirement for folate.

Selenium is an essential mineral needed to support the immune system and thyroid gland. The minimum daily recommended amount is small (only 55 micrograms) and is best acquired through foods such as Brazil nuts, sunflower seeds, sardines, and garlic. Eating one large Brazil nut a day is likely enough to fulfill the body's requirement.

Adaptogens are compounds that support the body's ability to cope with stress. The roots and berries of the ashwagandha plant (*Withania somnifera*) have been used for centuries in Ayurvedic medicine. Through its antioxidant properties, ashwagandha is believed to have a wide range of health benefits from improving brain function, stress resilience, and disease resistance to protecting against cellular damage and promoting a healthy sexual and reproductive balance. It is especially rejuvenating for the endocrine and immune systems.

This herb is often given to women when the balance of stress hormones and health needs additional support. Let's say you have improved your gut health and are maintaining a healthy diet but need more support during stressful times. Taking ashwagandha can help lower stress and anxiety, as well as balance energy and vitality. The dosage can vary, but most benefits are found at 500–600 mg per day taken for at least a month.

Emerging Contributors

Integrative practitioners continue to search for interventions to help sufferers of fatigue and chronic health syndromes. Looking deep into the root cause and the body's processes for metabolism, detoxification, and inflammation can lead to better solutions. In addition, the science around genetic testing to help improve clinical outcomes is emerging as a potential intervention.

Genes and Epigenetics

You may have been taught that your genetics influence who you are and what diseases you may acquire as you age. Genetics play a role, but perhaps not as much as you think. In 2016, an international team of researchers surveyed blood samples from 210 sets of twins ranging in age from 8 to 82, focusing on white blood cells and other markers of immune strength. The researchers concluded that 58% of the immune system is almost completely determined by nongenetic factors that you can influence every day. This is called epigenetics, which literally means "above" or "on top of" genetics. It refers to external modifications to DNA that turn genes "on" or "off." These modifications do not change the DNA sequence, but instead they affect how cells "read" genes. So your genes set the stage, but your diet and lifestyle choices impact how your genes will express themselves. For example, exposure to toxic chemicals, diet, stress, exercise, and other environmental factors are capable of eliciting positive or negative epigenetic modifications with lasting effects on gene expression.

Genetic Testing

Understanding your individual genetic blueprint may guide you to make healthy choices. Genetic testing is in its infancy when it comes to clinical application. Many testing tools exist, but which one is the best and how do you choose? The best advice is to first know why you want to get genetic testing and then to work with a knowledgeable practitioner who has been trained in the science and the application of gene testing and who knows how to interpret the results. Remember, your genetic blueprint is not a determinant of inevitability. Your environment and lifestyle play a major role in how that blueprint shows up in your life.

From an integrative medicine perspective, let's consider the example of a woman suffering with fatigue who has a variant in the MTHFR gene. This is the gene that instructs the body to make the enzyme that breaks down the amino acid homocysteine. The complex metabolism of homocysteine within the body is highly dependent on cofactors, including folate (B_9), B_2, B_6, and B_{12}. If this enzyme is not present, homocysteine levels can rise and cause health problems. With a variant in the MRHFR, an active form of all the B vitamins like folate (as 5-MTHF), B_6 (as pyridoxal-5-phosphate), and B_{12} (as methyl cobalamin) may be required to maintain a healthy homocysteine level. Conventional medicine does not subscribe to the need for the more active form of the B vitamins; however, remember Amy from earlier in the chapter. After a genetic test that showed a methylation variant, she started on an active form of the B vitamins along with improving her gut health; after 2 months, her fatigue and IBS remarkably improved. This may not have been the whole story in Amy's health recovery; however, from her perspective, healing occurred with these lifestyle modifiers.

HEALING SYSTEMS

If all these dietary suggestions and genetic information seem too overwhelming to start on your own, we recommend you seek professional support. Functional medicine physicians and naturopaths are skilled in multiple approaches to counteract your fatigue and improve your health. These practitioners are often fee-for-service and not covered by insurance. However, funds from a flexible spending account can be used to see a practitioner of your choice outside the conventional medical insurance system.

What Is Functional Medicine?

The term *functional medicine* was coined in 1991 by Dr. Jeffrey Bland, founder of the Institute of Functional Medicine in Gig Harbor, Washington. Functional medicine is a patient-centered healing approach that looks at the whole person through a lens of causation rather than simply treating symptoms. This approach to health and healing focuses intentionally on the how and why of illness. With regard to fatigue, consider these questions: "In what ways do I experience fatigue? What might be the underlying causes of this condition?"

Functional medicine seeks to restore health by addressing the root causes of disease, or a condition such as fatigue, for each unique individual. It looks closely at the myriad interactions that cause chronic disease, including genetics, social determinants, and environmental and lifestyle factors. Using scientific principles and advanced diagnostic testing (blood, stool, saliva, and genetic testing), along with addressing digestion, nutrition, hormone balance, stress reduction, and other self-care measures, functional medicine can restore balance in the body's primary physiological processes that lead to lifelong, optimal health.[4]

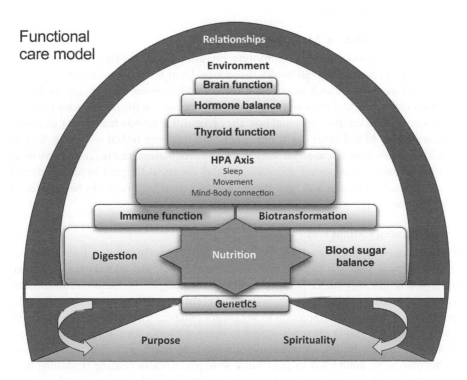

Illustration courtesy of Laura Sandquist.

What Is Naturopathic Medicine?

Naturopathic medicine is a "whole-systems" form of medicine that emphasizes prevention and individualized treatment of disease. This school of medical philosophy and practice centers on assisting the body's innate ability to establish, maintain, and restore health. The naturopath's role is to facilitate and augment this process, to identify and remove obstacles to health and recovery. It uses many modalities, including herbal medicine, acupuncture, osteopathy, nutrition, homeopathy, and lifestyle counseling, to address the underlying cause of disease. Fatigue or low energy is a common condition that requires attending to the root cause. Naturopathy provides natural therapies to encourage the individuals' inherent self-healing process.

Licensed naturopathic doctors (NDs) attend a 4-year, graduate-level naturopathic medical school. They are educated in all the same basic sciences as an MD, and they also study holistic and nontoxic approaches to therapy, emphasizing preventing disease and optimizing wellness. Their ability to practice is determined by state law, which varies from state to state. There are naturopaths, referred to as "traditional naturopaths," who are distinguished by having learned through other means, such as experientially from other healers/practitioners or via online courses. They may have extensive knowledge and skills but are not licensed or registered by a state or national accrediting board.

What Is Environmental Medicine?

Grave warnings about climate reality turn our attention to the fatigue of our planet and its effect on our personal health. Emerging from this climate urgency is environmental medicine, which examines ailments and diseases that are caused by the external environment. Environmental medicine focuses on the interactions between risk factors in the environment and how they jeopardize human health. For example, exposure to mold and other environmental toxins has been linked to chronic fatigue syndrome.[5] Environmental physicians focus on recognizing, treating, and preventing illnesses caused by exposure to biological and chemical triggers in air, food, and water. Consider whether and how these environmental factors might be sources of your fatigue.

What Is Energy Medicine?

Fatigue can be a complicated matter that affects many body systems. Even after you have improved your gut health, made dietary changes, and added essential nutrients, you might still suffer from low energy and fatigue. In these circumstances, you may consider consulting with an energy practitioner. Energy healing is a gentle, noninvasive therapeutic approach to regaining balance. This holistic practice activates the body's subtle energy systems to remove blocks. Breaking through these blocks stimulates the body's inherent ability to heal itself, providing a way for you to become more connected to your body wisdom. Ancient healing traditions have different names for energy, including *prana* (Hindu), *ruah* (Hebrew), and *qi* or *chi* (Chinese).

Energy Therapies and Techniques

Reiki is an energy healing practice that originated in Japan. The term comes from the Japanese words *rei*, meaning universal, and *ki*, which means vital life force energy that flows through all living things. Practitioners place their hands lightly on or just above the person's body, with the goal of directing energy to reduce stress and promote relaxation. This approach is based on the belief in an energy that supports the body's innate or natural healing abilities.

Healing Touch is an energy therapy that uses gentle hand techniques to help restore balance to the patient's energy field and accelerate the healing of the body, mind, and spirit. It is based on the belief that human beings are fields of energy that are in constant interaction with others and the environment. The goal of Healing Touch is to purposefully use the energetic interaction between the Healing Touch practitioner and the patient to restore harmony to the patient's energy system.

Reiki and Healing Touch are now part of patient care systems in many hospitals in the United States. Because of the effective results seen over recent years, energy healing has been actively researched for its benefits. There are training programs for individuals to become certified practitioners in this art of healing.

Within the field of energy healing are emerging techniques that some health practitioners use to identify subtle energy changes. *Muscle testing*, also known as applied kinesiology or manual muscle testing, is one of them. This gentle art of muscle monitoring is used to identify and treat imbalances in the body and has been likened to a kind of body biofeedback. For example, a practitioner may ask a question and see if the muscle gives away or gets weaker; this indicates a yes or no response. Although conventional medicine is not used to asking the body directly to respond to questions, many alternative practitioners feel that this approach reveals their patient's innermost voice. It helps the practitioner find the source of dysfunction in the body, such as fatigue.

Another tool is *electrodermal screening*, which uses an electronic device to measure a network of energy channels along the body's meridians. Meridian points, some of which correlate to the acupuncture points, are used to test body responses. Different organs are associated with each meridian point, and health problems are believed to manifest themselves as energetic disturbances in the associated meridian points. The screening procedure is done by measuring electrical resistance of the patient's skin when touched by a probe. The device contains a low-voltage source and registers the flow of current, determining the cause of disease by detecting an "energy imbalance." This tool might be helpful in getting at the root causes of your fatigue (eg, allergies, heavy metal toxicity, hormonal and enzyme deficiencies, vitamin and mineral imbalances) and in identifying which remedies to use, such as acupuncture, dietary changes, and/or vitamin supplements. There is a lot of debate on the validity of these screening tools/devices, but you may see them used by some alternative practitioners.

Most postmenopausal women have learned over the years that gut and health go hand in hand, yet may only be vaguely aware of the connection between the gut and fatigue. We believe that having a better understanding of *why and how* your gut responds to what you ingest—from food to external toxins—will help you choose holistic pathways to boost and sustain your energy.

PATHWAYS TO ENHANCE RESILIENCE

Self-Knowing: What do you notice about your level of energy? Is fatigue an issue in your life?

Self-Compassion: You need not accept fatigue as a way of life. In your efforts to gain more vitality, you can go at your own pace.

Self-Advocacy: What new strategies might you choose to enhance vitality? Do you need to reach out for more help?

CATHERINE'S PATHWAY

This chapter kind of stopped me in my tracks. I had no idea that fatigue can be such a complicated matter. The section on the gut really got my attention. I now better understand the "why" behind how foods and beverages can affect my system and energy flow. I am making adjustments to what I ingest food-wise but, truth be told, the decrease in my consumption of red wine will be quite modest.

Frankly, fatigue has not been a recent issue for me, since I "retired" from my full-time, all-consuming work as college faculty. I still engage in projects that require considerable brain energy, collaboration with others, and deadlines. I have figured out a few things that help keep my energy flowing. I usually get 8 hours of restful sleep each night. My chronic pain is at a manageable level through weekly workouts with my personal trainer (since 2007), regular exercise, and nonaddictive medication. Given that my home is now my office, I am creating an environment that gives me more aesthetic pleasure and a sense of calm. I am still working toward a better balance of work and play, of activity and rest, of being with myself and with others.

Over the years, I have tried many kinds of effective modalities and will likely try new ones. For sure, I with stick with acupuncture, healing touch, and personal training. These modalities offer me calm and energy—just the combination that suits me best.

9 Weight Concerns
Nourish Your Body

It is a rare woman who declares that she is at a good weight and satisfied with her body image. Weight is the #1 concern women typically express when asked about their health. "I know I need to lose weight, but I just can't." "I have tried every diet, and I just keep gaining weight." "I exercise every day, and I haven't lost a pound." Even women who would be considered slender often say, "I just have to get rid of this belly fat."

Weight dissatisfaction is a dominant stressor for many women that often does not dissipate with age. When you see an older woman with a prominent stomach or a plump grandmother caring for her grandchild, do you think she is content with those extra pounds? Most likely, not! Our desires, self-image, and passions do not fade away as we age. In fact, our concerns about weight can become more pronounced, even obsessive. Body weight is an emotionally charged matter and remains highly stigmatized in our culture. Our attention needs to shift away from "pounds to lose" to instead focus on healthy behaviors and health promotion.

Many of us became teens in the 1960s when weight loss was becoming commercialized and a popular topic in household conversations. For example, Carolyn's mother, a baker of wonderful bread, pies, and pastries, was always struggling to lose weight.

> *My mother was a founding member of Take Off Pounds Sensibly (TOPS). When talking about slow, sustainable weight loss, she would say, "If you think losing a pound a week is nothing, just hang a pound of butter on each hip and tell me that is nothing!" Whenever she was offered a serving of dessert, my mother repeated this saying: "No thank you, I have had ample sufficiency; more would be superciliously redundant as I am quite scrupulous about becoming too corpulent." She and her sister wrote that phrase in their early teens while trying to keep their weight in check. That was in the 1920s, so weight preoccupation is clearly not a new phenomenon.*

The baby boomers among us might remember the model Twiggy who came on the scene in the 1960s with her pencil-thin body, short skirts, and pixie-cute features. Some of us wanted to look just like this culture icon. Images like hers—and many others that followed—in magazines and on television have contributed to a cadre of dysfunctional thinking and behaviors around food.

A reality of aging, for many of us, is putting on weight. On average, women gain 1.5 pounds (0.7 kg) per year in their 50s and 60s, independent of initial body size or race/ethnicity.[1] These added pounds have to do with factors related to loss of estrogen, mood disorders, sleep disturbance, and, most significantly, changes in metabolism. Unless you are a woman who can still eat like you did in your 20s, you likely are dealing with the tensions between acceptance and intervention. What "natural

DOI: 10.1201/9781003250968-11

aging" changes are you willing to live with? How intentionally do you want to interrupt weight gain through new habits, such as diet and exercise?

Disordered Eating

Research dispels the myth that older women don't struggle with their self-image like younger women do. In a 2006 study of 1,000 women 60–70 years old, 80% controlled their body weight and 60% were unsatisfied with their bodies. In a 2012 study of women older than 50, 70% were trying to lose weight and 13% showed symptoms of an eating disorder.[2-3]

Disordered eating refers to a spectrum of irregular eating behaviors or habits that may or may not signal an actual eating disorder. An eating disorder is a more serious condition that disrupts your life and affects your health in numerous ways. Eating disorders can affect women of all ages and do not spare the aging woman. Anorexia nervosa, bulimia, and binge eating can affect women in midlife and later. What we don't know is whether older women with an eating disorder suffered from an untreated eating disorder in the past that may have gone into remission and resurfaced later in life, or if the disorder first appeared later in life. We do know that eating disorders have increased to the point that in America, 78% of deaths due to anorexia occur among older adults, not the young.[4]

Women seek treatment while in different phases of disordered eating, and addressing these issues is imperative before weight loss can be achieved and optimal weight maintained.

> *Heidi had been in treatment briefly during her teens for binge eating and admitted that, at the age of 48, she continued to struggle. A beautifully poised woman, Heidi was married with two daughters and taught grade school. I was one of the few people who knew of her continued struggle with binge-purge eating, and I felt relieved that she would confide in me. Heidi felt guilty about her behavior, and many times we discussed the need to seek treatment. Although she occasionally made a minimal attempt to seek counseling, Heidi seemed completely resigned that her condition was hopeless. She had lived with disordered eating for so long that changing her thoughts and behavior seemed impossible.*

This may seem like a discouraging story, but Heidi was able to compartmentalize her eating disorder in a way that she could manage it. She enjoyed her work, family, and friends yet at times would binge-purge. She could acknowledge the unhealthy behavior but did not let it dominate her life. Heidi also knew where to reach out for help if the disorder became unmanageable. It's important to note that an eating disorder does not define the whole person; it is only one component, albeit a significant one, of a woman's life.

Obesity

On the spectrum of disordered eating, obesity is a national crisis in the United States. The incidence of obesity has increased dramatically over the past 20 years such that it is now considered to be an epidemic. According to the U.S. Centers for Disease

Weight Category	Body Mass Index (BMI)* (kg/m²)
Underweight	<18.5
Normal	18.5–24.9
Overweight	25.0–29.9
Obese	30–35
Morbid obesity (stage III, extreme obesity, or clinically severe obesity)	>35

* BMI is calculated as weight in kilograms divided by height in meters squared. You can calculate your own BMI by going online, searching for "BMI calculator," and entering your weight and height.

Control and Prevention, obesity now affects more than one-third of adults, with two-thirds of the adult population either overweight or obese.[5] Nearly two-thirds of women 40–59 years old and about three-fourths of women 60 and older are overweight, defined as a body mass index (BMI) of greater than 25 kg/m². Furthermore, almost half of the women in these age groups are obese, meaning a BMI of 30 kg/m² or greater. BMI is a useful tool but far from a perfect measurement because it does not distinguish between body fat and muscle weight, and it does not indicate an individual's overall health.

Here are some staggering statistics about women in the United States:[6]

- The prevalence of obesity in women 60 and older is 43.3%.
- Minority women, low-income women, and women who live in certain geographic regions are at a particularly high risk of obesity.
- African American and Hispanic women are twice as likely as their White counterparts to be overweight or obese.
- The medical care costs of obesity are almost $150 billion per year.

The World Health Organization defines obesity as "a chronic relapsing disease process with food as the primary agent." Both overweight and obesity are linked to chronic low-grade inflammation.[7] While researchers continue to look for the inflammatory mechanism, it is known that pro-inflammatory cytokines are released. These cytokines are thought to be at the core of the complications associated with diabetes, cardiovascular disease, and chronic pain conditions.

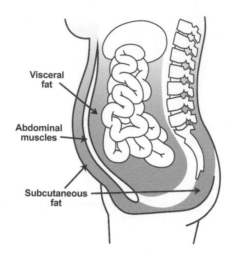

Illustration courtesy of Gary Johnson.

Abdominal Fat and Central Obesity

After menopause, women experience changes in the distribution of body fat. The proportion of fat to body weight tends to increase, and fat storage begins favoring the upper body over the hips and thighs. Even if you don't gain weight per se, your waistline can grow by inches as visceral fat pushes out against the abdominal wall.

There are two kinds of body fat: subcutaneous fat and visceral (intra-abdominal) fat.

Subcutaneous fat is the belly fat you can feel if you pinch excess skin and soft tissue around your middle. In most people, about 90% of body fat is subcutaneous, the kind that lies in a layer just beneath the skin.

Visceral fat accumulates in your abdomen in the spaces surrounding the liver, intestines, and other organs. It's also stored in the omentum, an apron-like flap of tissue that lies under the belly muscles and covers the intestines. Although visceral fat makes up only 10% of body fat, it is linked more strongly than subcutaneous fat to greater risk of serious health problems such as type 2 diabetes and heart disease. No matter what your body shape or BMI, excess belly fat isn't good for your health.

Metabolic Syndrome

Metabolic syndrome is a cluster of conditions that includes high levels of cholesterol and/or triglycerides, high fasting blood glucose, high insulin levels, high blood pressure, and central obesity. Although there is some variation in the definition, having a waist circumference of >35 inches plus two other risk factors meet the criteria for metabolic syndrome by the International Diabetes Federation.

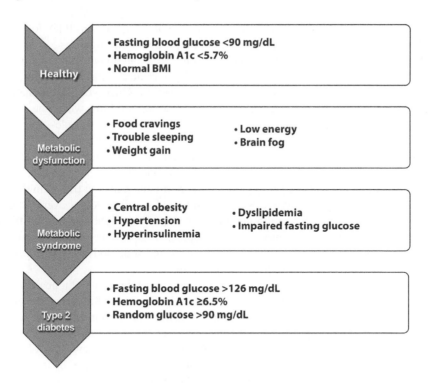

Healthy
- **Fasting blood glucose <90 mg/dL**
- **Hemoglobin A1c <5.7%**
- **Normal BMI**

Metabolic dysfunction
- **Food cravings**
- **Trouble sleeping**
- **Weight gain**
- **Low energy**
- **Brain fog**

Metabolic syndrome
- **Central obesity**
- **Hypertension**
- **Hyperinsulinemia**
- **Dyslipidemia**
- **Impaired fasting glucose**

Type 2 diabetes
- **Fasting blood glucose >126 mg/dL**
- **Hemoglobin A1c ≥6.5%**
- **Random glucose >90 mg/dL**

The Metabolic Spectrum

The term *insulin resistance* (also called insulin sensitivity) means that insulin, which is produced by the pancreas, can't transport glucose from the bloodstream into the body's cells. When insulin doesn't open the cell door to let glucose in, the cell is starved of glucose and sends the brain a signal that it is hungry. The glucose left sitting outside the cells increases the blood sugar level, which can lead to type 2 diabetes, and the extra glucose is stored as fat, which can lead to central obesity.

Why are we so concerned about metabolic syndrome? It is a strong predictor of a progressive chronic disease state, especially for heart health, stroke, and diabetes. Even though you may not have type 2 diabetes, you might be among the one-third of women who have metabolic syndrome or possibly a woman with mild metabolic dysfunction. Take a look and figure out where you are on the metabolic spectrum. The good news is that no matter where you fall on the spectrum, metabolic syndrome—especially when identified early—can be prevented or its impact can be reduced with lifestyle and dietary changes.

WEIGHT LOSS

As already noted, losing weight is the #1 issue for many women. Dieting is often the go-to strategy, despite the common refrain, "I may lose a few pounds, but they're back on in 6 months." In *Secrets from the Eating Lab*, Traci Mann, PhD, food psychologist and researcher, dispels a number of myths about dieting.[8]

Mann explains that the main reason diets don't work and do not lead to long-term weight loss is "because of your biology." When you reduce calories on a diet, your body goes into a survival mode against feeling starved. Once you go off the diet, your body wants to "fill up" again and gain back the weight. Plus, when you diet by calorie restriction, the weight you lose is about half fat and half muscle—but when the weight is regained, it is nearly all fat.

Body fat is an active part of the endocrine system, and it produces hormones that are involved in the sensation of hunger and fullness. One of these hormones is leptin. Often in obesity, the leptin signaling doesn't work properly, and so the brain doesn't get the clue to stop eating. We know that losing and gaining weight over and over ("yo-yo dieting") is bad for health and makes permanent weight loss more difficult because leptin and other hormones are disrupted. In addition, restricting calories leads to a physiological stress response, which means your body releases cortisol, which in turn leads to overeating and weight gain.

We also need to deal with many other barriers to weight loss and a healthy diet: cultural norms, emotional eating, lack of knowledge about healthy diets, lack of or difficult access to healthy foods, lack of satiety, lack of motivation, and more. A multitude of weight loss programs have hit the market over the years, including Weight Watchers, Nutrisystem, MyBistroMD, and Noom, to name just a few. The following are stories of three postmenopausal women who met the challenge of losing weight. Notice how they managed to modify their lifestyle and practice self-advocacy and self-care.

Claudia, at age 68, dropped from 161 to 139 pounds in 6 months. Determination was a big value in Claudia's life, and she walked daily, ate a plant-based diet, and made a mental commitment to lose weight. Claudia was planning to move to a warmer climate within the year, and she wanted to feel and look better.

Carrie, age 58, decided to try a program called SHAPE ReClaimed. In 2 months, she reduced from 182 pounds and a BMI of 32 kg/m² to 157 pounds with a BMI of 28 kg/m². The program involved weekly face time with a practitioner, a nanomolecular dietary supplement, a detailed dietary protocol, food planning, and the all-important accountability.

Lynn, age 74, lost weight on the Whole30® program. In 6 months, she reduced from 183 pounds and a BMI of 29 kg/m² to 155 pounds with a BMI of 24 kg/m². Her diet included foods that were anti-inflammatory with mostly protein, veggies, and some fruit. She avoided gluten, sugar, and dairy. Lynn reported feeling 10 years younger, along with reduced knee and joint pain. The Whole30 program encourages eliminating alcohol, sugar, grains, legumes, dairy, and additives from the diet. Recommendations include eating moderate portions of meat, seafood, and eggs; consuming lots of vegetables and some fruit; eating plenty of natural fats; and using herbs, spices, and seasonings rather than salt.

These women integrated exercise into their daily schedule and were able to sustain weight loss. Their stories illustrate that there is no one way to manage weight or one perfect diet plan for everyone. You need to figure out what will work for managing your weight in line with your body size and shape. We recommend this mindset: avoid the scale and focus on well-being.

BRIDGING THE GAP

Conventional medicine recognizes the epidemic of obesity and its impact on chronic disease. It also recognizes that the best way to address weight management is through a multidisciplinary approach based on behavioral modification, nutrition, physical activity, pharmacotherapy, and, when indicated, bariatric (weight-loss) surgery. The difficulty is that most physicians have minimal training in nutrition and limited time during a visit to discuss these interventions. Even more distressing is that negative views toward overweight and obese patients remain widespread among physicians, despite extensive scientific evidence that genetic and environmental factors often contribute to obesity. In a 2012 survey of 2,500 U.S. women, 69% reported feeling stigmatized by their doctors, and 52% endured recurring weight bias.[9] The problem is so pervasive that the American Medical Association and the American Academy of Pediatrics issued statements in 2017 emphasizing the importance of compassionate communication in an effort to ensure that overweight and obese patients are not stigmatized or shamed when seeking treatment for health issues.[10]

If you encounter these types of stigmatizing attitudes, this is definitely a time to call on your self-advocacy voice and ask for a referral to a nutritionist, a weight management clinic, or other resources. You deserve a more compassionate and integrative approach to weight loss.

INTEGRATIVE STRATEGIES

FOOD FACTORS

Over the decades, many attempts have been made to explain the biology behind weight management. In his 1996 best seller *Eating Right 4 Your Type*, Dr. Peter D'Adamo, a naturopathic physician, theorized that blood type was closely tied to the ability to digest certain types of foods and that the proper diet would improve digestion and help maintain ideal body weight.[11] Some individuals found this approach to eating helpful. Although there has never been any evidence to link blood type with the ability to make better food choices, the important takeaway is to understand how your body responds to foods and this differs for each person.

Another hypothesis is that food allergens are a significant contributing factor to obesity because they trigger systemic inflammation. In a 2020 study in which food allergens were identified in 237 foods, the elimination of the food allergens combined with aerobic-surge exercise yielded significant changes in weight, body fat percentage, and BMI.[12]

It is not a new concept that certain foods have harmful effects on the body. For example, consider the emerging knowledge about the underdiagnosis of gluten intolerance and celiac disease discussed in Chapter 8. Another problematic food is sugar, which is found in abundance in packaged and processed foods. Children most often develop the unhealthy habit of consuming a diet high in sugar, which can result in many detrimental health outcomes, including mood dysregulation, weight gain, and type 2 diabetes. When the habit of a high-sugar diet is carried into adulthood, we see chronic, often lifelong, health problems.

Consider what foods might be triggering your health outcomes. Is it that sugar-filled caramel roll that causes your knees to ache? Does a glass of milk in the morning result in constipation or diarrhea? The symptoms are often subtle, making food triggers hard to identify. That is why different laboratories perform food-sensitivity testing to identify potential triggers. We are not suggesting that this is the magic solution to weight loss or the ability to sustain good health. Rather, we want you to reflect on the possibility that some food may be triggering inflammation and adverse health conditions for you. Nourishing the body with nutrient-dense foods and high-quality natural foods is essential to support your well-being.

EPIGENETICS VERSUS GENETICS

You may wonder, "How much do my genes have to do with my body shape and size?" Your *genetics* is your DNA blueprint. In contrast, *epigenetics* is how your environment and behaviors can influence which of your genes are turned on or off and how the genes in your DNA are expressed. Genes can be activated or silenced by many factors, like what you eat, how you move, and how you manage your stress and exposure to environmental toxins. Because each of us starts with a unique DNA composition, what works for you will be different from what works for someone else. You know those women who can eat all they want and not gain weight? They likely have a genetic makeup that helps them to maintain that weight range. People are different when it comes to their ability to lose weight; some shed pounds quickly, while others have bodies that are more resistant to weight loss. Recent studies suggest that certain genetic variants may influence how you metabolize food and how that affects weight gain and obesity.

One gene receiving considerable attention is the apolipoprotein E *(APOE)* gene, which is found on chromosome 19 and is believed to confer risk factors for cardiovascular disease, Alzheimer disease, and obesity. The *APOE* gene has three common variants: E2, E3, and E4. The *APOE3* genotype is considered normal, found in about 60% of the general population. The *APOE4* genotype has been ascribed to unfavorable health outcomes such as weight gain and obesity.

You might hear a woman say, "The reason I am gaining weight is that I have the fat gene, *APOE4*." There may be some truth to this, but it is neither the whole story nor her destiny. You may have a predisposition for weight gain, but it is not inevitable. There are many strategies to counteract your genotype. If you come from a long line of overweight people, or you know you have the *APOE4* gene, you don't have to accept that you're doomed to obesity. The physical ability to lose, gain, or maintain a healthy weight varies considerably among individuals. Research in nutrigenomics and genomics testing is growing, and more knowledge of genetic variants may be able to guide you in selecting the best foods to eat for weight management.

Nourishment

The quote from Emily Maroutian, award-winning writer, poet, and philosopher is a favorite: "You're not stuck. You're just committed to certain patterns of behaviors because they helped you in the past. Now those behaviors have become more harmful than helpful." Some say that you just need to change your behavior, and you will get better results. However, we know from the *immunity to change* model (Chapter 3) that behaviors often are deeply embedded in beliefs. When your beliefs are framed as positive intentions, they can direct your behaviors toward your desired outcome. Or you could start the sequence by "acting as if," whereby you do the behaviors with the hope that they will align with, or get in line with, your beliefs. Either way, beliefs and behaviors are intertwined and need to be reconciled before an integrated weight management plan can be optimized.

Guidance and Support

Making choices about meal plans and food options can become overwhelming. We recommend consulting with a dietitian or nutritionist, professionals who can make the process more manageable. As you consider the options, keep in mind this fundamental question: what inhibits you from making the shift you know you need to make to change your dietary habits?

Functional dietitians or *nutritionists* are trained in the fundamental principles of whole-foods nutrition, particularly the concept of "food as medicine." Educational requirements differ for dietitians versus nutritionists, which has created confusion for patients. Here's what you should know about these practitioners. A *dietitian* is an expert in dietetics, a branch of knowledge concerned with diet and its effects on health. A dietitian will commonly work with patients to alter their nutrition based on a medical condition and/or individual goals. A registered dietitian (RD) has to complete at minimum a bachelor's degree in nutrition and dietetics and pass a national exam for certification. A *nutritionist* is a more general term that can apply to individuals with a variety of certifications and training. In the United States, the title "nutritionist" can be applied to anyone who offers general nutritional advice. Nutritionists are not as regulated as dietitians, yet many nutritionists have advanced degrees and have passed nutritionist certification boards. For example, a holistic nutritionist who specializes in functional nutrition may sit for the certification exam administered by the Holistic Nutrition Credentialing Board.

A nutritional consult typically begins with an in-depth evaluation to assess your diet and other lifestyle factors that may contribute to weight gain such as poor sleep patterns, limited physical activity, and life stressors. With this information, the nutritionist will work with you to identify opportunities for change. This doesn't always mean starting a diet. It could mean identifying and making one adjustment in your life that could impact your health. The care you get will be individualized for you.

The next step is formulating a plan that is suited to your specific needs. For instance, if you don't have time to cook and shop, options could include using a meal service that delivers healthy food to your door or receiving instructions on food selection when eating out. If you eat because of stress, the nutritionist will work with you to identify the underlying reasons for eating urges and strategies for managing them.

Seeking out a *health coach, integrative health coach,* or *well-being coach* is another approach to help you make behavior changes to improve your health and well-being. This coaching practice helps you identify your goals or desires, recognize where you are in a change process, leverage your strengths and assets, and determine what resources and support you need to achieve optimal well-being. This emerging profession of health coaching approaches wellness from a holistic perspective. Each woman is viewed as intrinsically whole and the ultimate expert in her own healing journey. Health coaching is being offered in a wide range of venues, including hospitals, clinics, community health and fitness facilities, corporations, educational institutions, and private practices.

Food as Medicine

The National Institutes of Health is leading efforts to advance the field of *precision nutrition* as the best strategy to catalyze nutrition science and related fields. The aim is to create meaningful, clinically relevant dietary solutions for both individuals and populations. The acknowledgment of "food as medicine" will increase our understanding of the therapeutic relationships among food, medications, and a wide range of health conditions and diseases.

When it comes to eating plans, most of us were brought up with the model "calories in versus calories out." The basic notion is that to maintain a stable weight, the number of calories you eat needs to match the number of calories you expend. Therefore, to lose weight, you need to eat fewer calories and/or burn more calories. We have been taught that getting our calories through carbohydrate, protein, or fat doesn't matter because a calorie is a calorie.

However, there is more to the story. The saying "Let food be thy medicine and medicine be thy food" hearkens back to Hippocrates, the father of medicine. This quote, though thousands of years old, acknowledges the importance of healthy foods and how the nutrients in various foods help with satiety and energy levels and even provide healing properties. Even if we were to concede that "calories in versus calories out" is the key to weight loss, it is the macronutrient composition that carries vital metabolic benefits for overall health and can't be ignored. Also, remember that the problem is not solved with a singular focus on what and how much to eat but rather why, where, and with whom you eat.

Mindful Eating

Attention to mindful eating is the first step in weight management. This means taking the time to mindfully enjoy your food by sitting and doing nothing else at mealtimes except eat. No smartphone, no computer, no television. Not even a book or magazine. Eating should not be on your multitasking agenda. And take note that eating while engaged in other activities often leads to mindless overeating.

A healthy digestive system is a powerful part of lifelong health, and mindful eating is the first step. Mindful eating allows your gastrointestinal tract to properly digest your food. Here are some tips for mindful eating:

- First, remember that spending a little extra time in the kitchen to prepare nutritious, whole foods that you enjoy will pay off big dividends for your overall health.
- While you are preparing food and eating your meal, take time to enjoy the food's aroma. Engaging your sense of smell stimulates your body to produce digestive enzymes.
- Before you eat, pause for a moment of gratitude.
- Concentrate on eating your meal without other distractions.
- Take time to chew your food. Chewing releases saliva, which is another source of needed digestive enzymes.
- Eating is a social activity, and you will likely engage in conversations during your meal. However, keep the dialogue from becoming heated or stressful. Save the fiery debate for another time.

Taking these simple steps to a mindful approach to eating will likely improve your digestion as well as help modify the amount you eat. You may find additional benefits to mindful eating, as Tracy discovered.

Tracy, age 60, came to my office expressing a desire to lose weight and concerns over not feeling well with considerable fatigue. She felt her digestion was poor, with constant gas and bloating. She felt highly irritable, had put on 10 pounds over the last couple of years, and struggled with headaches. As a small business owner, she commuted into town three or four times a week to manage her store. Tracy was overwhelmed and unsure what to do to improve her digestion and lose some weight. We discussed practicing mindful eating, trying a trial of a 30-day elimination diet, adding probiotics, avoiding trigger foods, and addressing some of her life stressors. She acknowledged that she needed to make changes in her life and agreed to start some of these strategies.

During a follow-up visit 3 months later, Tracy said she was feeling so much better. I asked her which of the strategies seemed to make the most difference for her, and she said, "Actually, I did just one thing. I ate mindfully. I sat down every morning for breakfast with my husband. By taking the time to eat and talk with him, I rediscovered how much I really like and enjoy him. We reconnected with good conversations, something we hadn't done in years. Also, when I went to work during the week, I started having lunch with my employees. We closed the store for half an hour and sat together to eat and talk. I realized how lucky I was to have such good people working with me, and everyone felt more relaxed and less stressed. Wow, the power of mindful eating has changed my life."

The Three Main Nutrients

Carbohydrates, protein, and fat are the three main nutrients, digested into simpler compounds for our bodies to use and function. Carbohydrates (starches and sugars) are used for energy in the form of glucose. Proteins are broken down into amino acids, which are used to build muscle and to make other proteins that the body needs. Fats are used for energy after they are broken down into fatty acids.

Carbohydrates are the body's main source of energy because they are the primary source of fuel for your brain's high energy demands. After a meal, sugar is converted

Nutrient	Sources	How Used
Carbohydrates (sugars and starches) *Simple carbs:* sugars that are easy to digest (eg, glucose and fructose) *Complex carbs:* starches that take longer to digest	• Breads • Grains • Fruits • Vegetables • Milk and yogurt • Foods with sugar (eg, soda) • High-fructose corn syrup	Broken down into glucose, used to supply energy to cells. Extra is stored in the liver or converted into fat stores.
Protein *Complete:* contains all the essential amino acids *Incomplete:* missing one or more amino acids	• Meat • Seafood • Legumes/beans • Nuts and seeds • Eggs • Milk products • Vegetables	Broken down into amino acids, used to build muscle and to make other essential proteins.
Fats *Unsaturated:* liquid at room temp *Saturated:* solid at room temp	• Oils • Butter • Egg yolks • Animal products	Broken down into fatty acids to make cell linings and hormones. Extra is stored in fat cells.

into glucose and sent into the bloodstream. This signals the pancreas to release insulin into the bloodstream. Insulin helps glucose enter the body's cells to be used for energy. If all the glucose is not needed for energy, some of it is stored in fat cells and in the liver as glycogen.

In a healthy individual, on a well-balanced diet, glucose moves from the bloodstream into the cells, and the blood glucose level returns to a normal range between meals. However, as we age, *insulin resistance* commonly develops. This means that the cells become less and less responsive to the signals of insulin and glucose. Glucose is not able to enter cells, so the cells do not have the energy they need. The signal sent to the brain is to eat more sugar, which leads to a cycle of overeating due to carb cravings and low energy. In addition, when glucose cannot enter cells, the glucose level rises in the bloodstream and can result in type 2 diabetes.

What is the difference between a simple and a complex carbohydrate? Complex carbohydrates contain longer chains of sugar molecules than simple carbohydrates. The longer chains mean complex carbs take longer to break down, and so your blood glucose level is more stable. Keeping a more stable blood glucose reduces food cravings.

So a good first step is to reduce your intake of simple carbohydrates. You can do this by eating plenty of fiber-rich fruits and vegetables, whole-grain carbohydrates in moderation, lean protein, and a moderate amount of healthy fats. If you increase your intake of healthy fats and decrease your carbohydrate intake low enough, your body will burn fat instead of sugar for energy. Fat will be converted into compounds called ketones, which are a powerful energy source. This is the concept behind a ketogenic or low-carb diet.

Fats are nutrients that give you energy. In a typical diet, 20%–35% of the calories come from fats. Fats help with the absorption of vitamins and minerals and are needed to build membranes and protective layers around cells and nerves. Fats also help with blood clotting, inflammation, and muscle movement. Fats are either saturated or unsaturated. Most foods with fat have both types, but usually there is more of one kind of fat than the other.

Unsaturated fats are considered "good" fats in the right ratio. You can tell that a fat is unsaturated if it is liquid at room temperature. Unsaturated fats can be monounsaturated or polyunsaturated. The best-known product containing monounsaturated fats is olive oil (think the Mediterranean diet). Canola oil, peanut oil, avocados, and some nuts are other examples of monounsaturated fats. The two main types of polyunsaturated fats are omega-3 fatty acids and omega-6 fatty acids. Foods with omega-3 fatty acids include salmon, mackerel, sardines, and flaxseeds. Foods with omega-6 fatty acids include vegetable oils such as corn, safflower, soybean, sunflower, and walnut oil.

Saturated fats are solid at room temperature. They are primarily from animal food products, including red meat, whole milk, cheese, and coconut oil. The value of saturated fat is under considerable debate. We advise postmenopausal women to minimize their intake of saturated fats (unless your experience with a diet high in saturated fats has brought you success). Some women are successful with a ketogenic diet that is high in fat, but that is likely because they are sticking to a food regimen that is limited in calories and still satisfying.

Trans fats, or *trans fatty acids*, are of two types: naturally occurring and artificial. Naturally occurring trans fats are produced in the guts of some animals, and foods made from these animals (eg, milk and meat products) may contain *small* amounts of these fats. Artificial trans fats, which are partially hydrogenated, are what we encourage you not to eat. They were deemed unsafe by the FDA in 2015 because of their link to heart attacks and stroke; they can raise LDL (the bad) cholesterol and lower HDL (the good) cholesterol levels. To minimize your trans-fat intake, avoid all vegetable oils and margarines that list partially hydrogenated oil as an ingredient.

Protein is needed to build and maintain muscles, tendons, and ligaments, as well as the brain and other organs. Proteins are made from chains of amino acids. Because protein is not stored in the body like carbs and fats, it should be eaten at every meal. Consuming enough protein is important to prevent the loss of lean muscle mass that occurs naturally with age. Yet, half of women 71 and older fall short of eating the recommended amount of protein.

Protein needs tend to increase for women as they age, primarily because of the natural loss of skeletal muscle, which affects 10% of adults older than 50. Therefore, to maintain muscle mass, a healthy adult woman over 50 should consume 1–1.2 grams of protein per kg (0.45–0.55 grams per pound) of body weight per day. For example, an older woman who should weigh 150 pounds may need to eat ~80 grams (0.55 × 150) or more of protein daily. Physically active women will need more protein. Protein acts synergistically with exercise to increase muscle mass so that incorporation of both is essential to slow muscle loss.

Amount of Protein in Common Foods

Food Source	Protein (grams)
Peanut butter, 2 tablespoons	8
Nonfat milk, 1 cup	8.8
Eggs, 2 medium	11.4
Chicken leg	12.2
Cottage cheese, half cup (4 oz)	15
Turkey, 3 oz	26.8
Edamame, shelled, 1 cup	18.4

Proteins are either complete or incomplete. Complete proteins contain all the essential amino acids our bodies need. Incomplete proteins are missing one or more of the essential amino acids. Foods found in animals are complete proteins and include meat, poultry, fish, eggs, milk, cheese, and other dairy products. Unfortunately, many of these animal proteins are high in insulin-like growth factor 1, which can promote weight gain. That doesn't mean that you need to avoid animal protein altogether but, if possible, select free-range animal sources that limit antibiotics and growth hormones.

Another way to meet your protein needs is by eating more plant-based proteins. Although many plant-based proteins are incomplete proteins, they become complete proteins when mixed with certain other plant-based proteins, such as eating corn tortillas and beans together. Legumes (beans, lentils, peas), nuts, seeds, whole grains, and vegetables are examples of healthy foods that contain incomplete proteins. Soy, amaranth, quinoa, hemp seed, and chia are examples of complete proteins that are plant-based. Consider expanding your food choices by choosing more plant-based foods.

The Right Diet

Most postmenopausal women today have been raised with the standard American diet, which is typically high in carbohydrates and trans fats and includes lots of processed and fast foods. So, what is the right diet? We first need to understand that much of the confusion about the right foods and the right diet has become more problematic since the industrialization of food, especially with so many "fast, processed, and convenient" foods readily available.

Baby boomers have been subject to a failed experiment regarding processed foods. One example is what happened in 1953 when the Swanson corporation drastically overestimated how many turkeys people would buy that year. Left with a surplus of 260 tons of frozen birds, Swanson ordered thousands of metal trays and concocted a meal featuring pressed turkey, cornbread dressing and gravy, peas, and sweet potatoes. The frozen meal (TV dinner) sold for 98 cents and was an instant hit. This is just one example of how our diets have been influenced by the food industry that has provided us with processed, easy-to-prepare, and often inexpensive foods that are, unfortunately, nutrient deficient and often high in salt, fat, and sugar.

Eating convenient, processed foods has greatly contributed not only to the obesity epidemic but also to depriving us of adequate nourishment. Understanding how to choose healthy foods has become complicated and confusing. Information between food marketers and scientific studies is often conflicting. What is best: a low-fat diet, a low-carb diet, or a high-protein diet? Scientific evidence is still lacking. However, it's clear that the standard American diet can result in systemic inflammation and is not optimal for weight control.

We need to look at new approaches for nourishing our bodies. Michael Pollan, author of *Food Rules: An Eater's Manual*, provides simple, straightforward advice: "Eat food. Not too much. Mostly plants."[13] A plant-based diet is a good place to start because it avoids foods that trigger inflammation.

The concept of an *anti-inflammatory diet* has emerged as new research suggests that certain foods actually trigger inflammation, which causes chronic health conditions. There is no single "right" anti-inflammatory diet, but any such diet should avoid pro-inflammatory foods and provide the right balance of healthy proteins, carbs, and fats at each meal, including plenty of fresh fruits and vegetables, whole grains, and healthful fats. A vegetarian or vegan diet may be one option for people looking to reduce inflammation and lose weight. The authors of a 2019 review analyzed data from 40 studies and concluded that people who eat a vegetarian-based diet are likely to have lower levels of various inflammatory markers.[14–15]

The following foods increase inflammation and need to be limited in your diet:

- Sugary beverages (eg, sugar-sweetened drinks, fruit juices)
- Refined carbs (eg, white bread, white pasta)
- Desserts (eg, cookies, candy, cake, ice cream)
- Processed meat (eg, hot dogs, bologna, sausages)
- Processed snack foods (eg, crackers, chips, pretzels)
- Trans fats, found in foods with partially hydrogenated ingredients
- Alcohol (excessive consumption)

Two well-established diets have been combined recently to form a new eating pattern called MIND—Mediterranean–DASH Intervention for Neurodegenerative Delay. The Mediterranean diet, which is associated with the traditional foods in countries like Italy and Greece, has proved to reduce inflammatory biomarkers such as C-reactive protein and interleukin-6. The focus of the DASH diet (Dietary Approaches to Stop Hypertension) is to help lower high blood pressure. It emphasizes foods that are lower in sodium and rich in potassium, magnesium, and calcium.

The MIND diet is especially good for heart health; for individuals with metabolic syndrome, high triglycerides, diabetes, prediabetes, and/or hypertension; and for postmenopausal women. It has also been shown to slow cognitive loss and support weight loss. A significant improvement of the MIND diet over the DASH diet is the high-fiber content (43 grams) through the higher intake of fruits and vegetables.

Mediterranean diet	• Vegetables, fruits, nuts, seeds, legumes, potatoes, whole grains, breads, herbs, spices, fish, seafood, and extra virgin olive oil • Moderate amounts of poultry, eggs, cheese, and yogurt • Limited amounts of red meat and dairy • Moderate amount of red wine (1 glass a day) *Nutrient ratio: 50% carbs, 15% protein, 35% fat*
DASH diet	• Fruits and veggies, including low-fat dairy products, whole grains, fish, poultry, and nuts • Moderate amounts of lean meat, fish, and poultry *Nutrient ratio: 55% carbs, 18% protein, 33% fat*
MIND diet	• More heart-healthy fats • Less refined starchy or added-sugar foods *Nutrient ratio: 38% carbs, 26% protein, 36% fat*

We are all looking for the right diet for our body constitution. Research is making progress to find markers that will help you choose the best foods to eat. New apps are becoming available to guide you in meal selection. Diet ID™ is a digital toolkit that provides dietary assessment and management with an innovative, visual approach to optimizing health. Dr. David Katz, who developed this evidenced-based application, says it is like a GPS: it tells you where you are starting from, where to go, and how to get there by generating results and individual plans in real time. New programs and products come on the market all the time, so before you make a commitment, be sure to research capabilities and read the reviews of the ones that appeal to you.

Glycemic Index and Glycemic Load

The glycemic index has come in and out of fashion since it was first created in the 1980s. The glycemic index is not a diet plan but a tool—such as calorie counting or carb counting—to guide choosing foods that promote weight loss and prevent diseases related to obesity such as diabetes and cardiovascular disease.

The *glycemic index* of a food indicates how much that food *increases blood glucose levels*. A low glycemic index is 1–55, medium is 56–69, and high is 70 and up. Lower values are a guide to helping you make healthier food choices. For example, the glycemic index of an English muffin made with white flour is 77, whereas that of a whole-wheat English muffin is 45. In general, foods with a low glycemic index are digested and absorbed relatively slowly, and those with high values are absorbed quickly.

One limitation of the glycemic index is that it doesn't reflect how much of a food you eat. To address this problem, the concept of *glycemic load* was developed. Glycemic load indicates the *change in blood glucose levels* when you eat a typical serving of the food. A low glycemic load is 1–10, medium is 11–19, and high is 20 and up. A few examples: a large carrot has a glycemic load of 2, a medium apple of 6, a large banana of 14, and a small box of raisins scores 20.

Glycemic index and glycemic load can be effective tools that may help you make better decisions about what foods can help manage your blood sugar and weight. Having a chart listing the glycemic index and glycemic load of common foods is very helpful when starting to use this tool. Many charts of foods can be found online.

Meal Plans

We have all been exposed to a plethora of dietary options over the years. Here, we present four common diets for you to compare and contrast: the standard American diet, a ketogenic (or "keto") diet, the Paleo diet, and a vegan diet, all at approximately 2,000 calories per day.

The *standard American diet* has historically been followed by most Americans. It is characterized by high intake of red meat, processed meat, chicken, refined grains, and pre-packaged foods. Most calories come from grain products, such as bread, rolls, bagels, pizza, and desserts. The diet is high in sodium, sugar, animal fats, and hydrogenated vegetable oils.

The *ketogenic diet* focuses on foods that provide a lot of healthful fats, adequate amounts of protein, and very few carbohydrates (no more than 20–25 grams per day). The purpose is to kick your body into ketosis, a metabolic state that forces your body to burn fat rather than carbs.

Sample Meal Plans for Four Common Diets

	Standard American	Keto	Paleo	Vegan and Vegetarian
Nutrient ratio	Carbs 45%–65% Protein 10%–35% Fat 20%–35%	Carbs 5%–10% Protein 20%–25% Fat 70%	Carbs 30% Protein 30% Fat 40%	Carbs 40%–65% Protein 20%–30% Fat 20%–25%
Breakfast	Bowl of corn flakes with 1% milk, orange juice	Two fried eggs, tomato slices, coffee with cream	Eggs and vegetables fried in coconut oil, piece of fruit	Oatmeal with fruit and flaxseeds
Snack	Low-fat yogurt	Full-fat cottage cheese topped with pine nuts	Beef jerky	Apple with a few walnuts
Lunch	Roast beef sandwich with American cheese, mayonnaise, and tomato, apple slices	Spinach salad with grass-fed burger, cheese, and avocado	Chicken salad with olive oil, handful of nuts	Grilled veggie and hummus wrap with sweet potato fries
Snack	Popcorn	Roasted, salted almonds	Guacamole with vegetables	½ cup nonfat plain Greek yogurt (soy yogurt if vegan) with blueberries
Dinner	Chicken breast fried in vegetable oil, baked potato, green beans and carrots, dinner roll	Grilled salmon, broccoli with butter	Salmon fried in butter, vegetables, some berries	Butternut squash and black bean tostadas

The *Paleo diet* typically includes lean meats, fish, fruits, vegetables, nuts, and seeds—foods that in the past (the Paleolithic era) could be obtained by hunting and gathering. This plan focuses on whole, unprocessed foods and eliminates added sugars, grains, legumes, and dairy.

Vegetarian and vegan diets primarily differ in that vegetarians avoid only meat, while vegans avoid all animal-sourced products, including eggs, honey, and dairy.

Maybe one of these diets has already resonated with you and been helpful for weight management. But if you are still left asking, *"What meal plan is best for me?"* you may be interested in the Postmenopausal Eating Plan, described in the next section.

Postmenopausal Eating Plan (PEP)©

The PEP is a meal plan that Carolyn formulated to help women manage their weight and find success with healthy eating habits. The PEP shifts your meal plan from the standard American diet to include less carbohydrates and more protein (eg, carbs 35%, protein 30%, and fat 35%). The reason for this is that postmenopausal women have a tightly regulated carbohydrate threshold below which we burn fat and lose weight. If carbohydrate intake exceeds this threshold, carbohydrate burning predominates, allowing fat to accumulate along with added pounds. For most postmenopausal women, a lower carbohydrate diet with adequate protein is the way to go.

First, understanding what is meant by high, moderate, low, and extremely low carbohydrates in a diet is essential for weight loss.

Now let's compare the standard American diet and the PEP.

Carbohydrate Intake	
Carbohydrate Level	Dietary Intake (grams per day)
High	>200
Moderate	100–200
Low	50–100
Extremely low	<50

	Standard American Diet	Postmenopausal Eating Plan
Carbs	60%	35%
Calories	900–1200	525–700
Grams	225–300	131–175
Protein	20%	30%
Calories	300–400	450–600
Grams	75–100	112–150
Fat	20%	35%
Calories	300–400	525–700
Grams	33–44	58–78

Note: Both diets based on 1,500–2,000 calories per day.
1 gram of carbohydrate = 4 calories, 1 gram of protein = 4 calories, and 1 gram of fat = 9 calories.

You can see that the standard American diet is a high-carb diet, which is *not* desirable for postmenopausal women. In contrast, the PEP is a moderate-carb diet and provides more protein. Remember that we need more dietary protein as we age because our bodies break down and use protein less efficiently. The higher fat allowance in the PEP also helps with feeling full or satisfied, and at least 50% of the fat should be from monounsaturated fatty acids (eg, olive oil).

An important step to success in the PEP diet is to know how many carbohydrates you are eating in a typical day. To do this, you'll need to keep a food diary for 1–3 days. If you have never counted carbohydrates, this will be a valuable exercise—and you may be shocked at what you'll learn!

Write down everything you eat and how you feel. Then figure out how many carbs you've eaten. Figuring out how many carbs are in a given food is easier than you may think. Carbs (as well as protein, fat, and other nutrients) are on the label of packaged food items. The carb content of fresh produce, meats, fish, and so on are easy to find online. You should now have an idea of how many carbs you have typically been eating in a day. Now eat a lower-carb diet (50–60 grams per day) for 1–3 days. Write down how you feel on this diet and compare it to how you felt before. You may be surprised by the difference this simple change in carbohydrate intake can make.

Sarah was a healthy 60 year old, 5 feet 4 inches tall and 140 pounds, with a healthy BMI of 24 kg/m². She wanted to get down to 130 pounds with a BMI of 22 kg/m², like she had been during her younger adult life. The extra 10 pounds she had put on, mostly around her belly, was not going away, despite her very healthy diet and daily exercise. I asked Sarah about how many grams of carbohydrates she ate in a typical day. She had no idea but knew she kept her daily calorie intake at about 1,500. I suggested she keep track of her carbohydrate intake for 2 or 3 days, and then aim for a low-carb intake of 100 grams/day with protein at each meal to total about 120 grams of protein per day. I advised her that by consuming too many carbs and too little protein she would find it nearly impossible to lose weight. Sarah seemed somewhat frustrated that I could not give her more suggestions on weight loss. However, since she had never intentionally counted her carbohydrate intake before, she said she would try this approach. When I saw Sarah for an unrelated problem 3 months later, she said, "Oh, by the way, I read about the low-carb diet you suggested, and it's really working for me—I've already lost 5 pounds! I had no idea that I was getting more than 300 grams of carbs a day. Now I stay at 100–150 and make sure I have some protein at each meal." Sarah's diet plan followed the recommended moderate amount of carbs in the PEP (100–200 grams per day) and helped her succeed in achieving and maintaining her desired weight.

As illustrated by Sarah's story, discovering the amount of carb intake that works for you and then committing to that as part of your diet plan may be what you need to do. Staying on a low-carb diet of 50–100 grams per day is difficult to sustain, but maintaining a carb intake of 100–200 grams per day is a more reasonable challenge and is consistent with the PEP.

Another important factor in making this work is to choose the right kind of carbohydrates, and plant-based carbohydrates are the way to go. You also need to eat adequate protein with every meal, a minimum of 3 oz (21 grams) at regular intervals throughout the day. Starting the day with a healthy protein breakfast will keep your metabolism running at an optimal level and prevent breakdown of muscle tissue.

Sample Daily Meal Plans

Breakfast	Coffee with soy creamer	Green tea with almond creamer
	2 eggs with 1 slice Ezekiel bread and 1 tbsp almond butter	Oatmeal with ½ cup yogurt, ½ cup blueberries, and chopped walnuts
Snack	1/3 cantaloupe	Apple with cheese or bell peppers in cheese wrap
Lunch	Spinach salad with 3 oz tuna and ½ cup cottage cheese	Mixed greens/peppers with dressing and ½ cup shelled edamame
Snack	½ avocado (guacamole) with a handful of corn chips or veggies	Hummus and carrots
Dinner	Salmon (3 oz) with roasted cauliflower and broccoli, ½ cup wild rice	Chicken breast with roasted zucchini with tomatoes, ½ cup black beans
	A glass of wine or hibiscus tea slightly sweetened	A glass of wine or hibiscus tea slightly sweetened

Note: Sample plans provide ~1,800 calories, 150 grams carbs, and 100 grams protein daily.
Use onions, mushrooms, garlic, and spices as desired. Pay attention to portion size.

During the weight-loss process, you want to preserve—not lose—lean body mass while getting rid of extra body fat. Eating adequate protein may be a challenge for some of you because we seem to be surrounded by carbohydrates. So, you may need to make an effort to seek out healthy plant-based sources of protein.

Keep in mind that the PEP is a pathway to manage weight, not a rigid meal plan. There is flexibility in your food choices, and finding out what works for you is part of the exploration. The balance of quality carbohydrates, protein, and fat along with calorie management is all part of the solution to ideal weight.

Realistic Goals

If you have a significant amount of weight to lose, it may be too discouraging to think about doing it all at once. Rather than zeroing in on a number, focus on making and sustaining healthy lifestyle changes. Often when talking to a woman about weight loss, she will say, "I want to lose 50 pounds" or "I want to get down to the weight I was before I was pregnant." Many times, her goal is to lose weight as quickly as possible. A more realistic, and less daunting, approach is to aim for a sustainable weight loss. Losing 1 pound a week would translate to a loss of 52 pounds in a year—an impressive achievement.

HEALING SYSTEMS AND APPROACHES

Fasting

Fasting is one of the most ancient, inexpensive, and powerful healing strategies known to humankind. Many cultures and religions have practiced some form of fasting—both as spiritual rituals and as ways to cleanse the body. In our current secular culture, intermittent fasting, also called "time-restricted eating," has recently become popular. In this eating pattern, you cycle between fasting, typically for 12–16 hours, and eating within a window of 8–12 hours. The hypothesis is that when you go into a state of fasting, especially for longer than 14 hours, you deplete the body of its glucose reservoir. After the glucose is depleted from reducing your calorie intake, your body starts to break down fat for energy.

Here are two popular intermittent fasting options, followed by a few pointers:

1. Eat normally for 5 days, and then eat 500 calories on each of the next 2 days.
2. Eat only during a window of 8–12 hours, which gives your body 12–16 hours of fasting daily. Start by eating your meals in a 12-hour window. Once this becomes easy, reduce your eating window to 10 hours and then to 8 hours if possible. During your fasting window, drink only noncaloric beverages such as purified water, teas, and black coffee.

- Caffeine intake in a fasted state increases your ability to burn fat. Because of this, caffeine can be used strategically to increase ketone levels and subdue hunger.
- Your first meal of the day should include both fiber and protein, so that you'll feel satisfied until your next meal.
- First thing in the morning (within an hour or two of waking up), drink 8–16 ounces of filtered water.
- Try the Postmenopausal Eating Plan with a 10-hour eating window (eg, first meal at 10 a.m., snack at 2 p.m., second meal at 6 p.m., snack at 8 p.m.).

Fasting can be effective if done wisely. But it is not for everyone, and it is not essential for a healthy, vital life. It is simply one option that may prove useful when it comes to sustainable weight management.

Exercise and Activity

Participating in some form of movement or activity every day is essential. An eye-opening article published in the *Journal of the American Medical Association* in March 2010 reported on a study that enrolled 34,000 women (average age 54.2 years old). The researchers examined which women were able to maintain their weight during the transition through menopause and beyond. The women who successfully maintained normal weight and gained fewer than 5 pounds (2.3 kg) over a 13-year period averaged approximately 60 minutes a day of moderate-intensity activity.[16] Although this amount of daily exercise isn't attainable or appealing for everyone, there is no question that exercise is a powerful lifestyle intervention. Even small amounts of physical activity, as little as 10 minutes at a time, are beneficial. In the recent book *In Praise of Walking: A New Scientific Exploration*, author Shane O'Mara reminds us of the many benefits of walking and encourages us to get out of our chairs and discover a happier, healthier, more creative self.[17]

PHYSICAL ACTIVITY = POTENT MEDICINE

- When losing weight, more physical activity increases the number of calories your body uses for energy or "burns off." Burning calories combined with reducing the number of calories you eat creates a calorie deficit that results in weight loss.
- Most weight loss occurs because of decreased caloric intake. However, the only way to *maintain* weight loss is to be engaged in regular physical activity.
- Most importantly, physical activity reduces risks of cardiovascular disease and diabetes beyond that resulting from weight loss alone.

———————

Even as you adopt healthy lifestyle strategies, the reality is that your physical body changes as you age. Subtle changes are more noticeable to you than to anyone else: morning aches and pains, a few more laugh lines, a bladder with a mind of its own. Other changes require you to modify your activity levels or take different supplements. The ultimate goal is to find your own healthy balance between body image and body acceptance. While your body can continue to serve you well as you age, you may need to adopt new patterns of being active. Eating well, exercising, and accepting yourself in whatever body shape or size you have are all essential elements of nourishing the body, mind, and spirit.

PATHWAYS TO NOURISH YOUR BODY

Self-Awareness: What is your image of your body? What are the messages that you internalize about your body? How do you talk about your body to yourself and others?

Self-Compassion: Acknowledge the tension between accepting yourself as you are, yet wanting to change your weight in some way.

Self-Advocacy: When you are ready to make some changes, what will you commit to doing? Where can you find the support you need to nourish your body?

———————

CATHERINE'S PATHWAY

Talking candidly about sexual health is easier for me than dealing with the topic of my weight. At age 18, I was 5'11" tall and weighed 135 pounds. I looked good in a bathing suit, dresses, and jeans alike. I biked, hiked, and canoed with vigor. As the years progressed, I put on weight. I sat too much in my professional work, took a triumph over the body approach to dealing with stress, and limited my physical activity because of chronic back pain. By the time I was postmenopausal, I was adding and losing the same 10 pounds, then it became 20 pounds. Now, at age 72, I am humbled to be one of those postmenopausal women who would do well to lose 40 pounds.

Clearly, it's time to make a firm commitment to reaching and maintaining a desirable weight. I am not lacking in knowledge about what and how much to eat or drink, what kind and how much exercise to do, and ways to engage in emotional and spiritual self-care. Yet, I admit to having an "immunity to change" mindset when it comes to consistently doing what's best for my physical body. I will continue to work with my personal trainer on core, strength, and balance; stock whole foods, especially those good for digestion; and ride my exercise bike daily, increasing the time incrementally. Living alone comes with many freedoms, but I need to be accountable, so I will look for a program or a person who can travel with me on my weight management journey.

10 Bone Health
Build Your Core

All of us want to remain active and agile as we age. Preserving our mobility requires addressing bone health. We want to emphasize the value of bone health through the lens of maintaining bone strength and bone density rather than focusing only on bone loss. Of course, osteopenia and osteoporosis are serious concerns for many postmenopausal women. Of the estimated 10 million Americans with osteoporosis, about 80% are women, and one in four women in the United States older than 65 has osteoporosis.[1–2] Osteoporosis causes bones to become porous and brittle—a condition that we can't see or feel. Without any obvious symptoms, often the first indication of osteoporosis is a bone fracture. For this reason, osteoporosis has been called "the silent epidemic."

How well do you know your own bones? Have you had a DXA scan to measure your bone health? If so, do you know your T-score? If you have low bone density, how will you build your bone strength to prevent osteoporosis? If you have osteoporosis, how will you stabilize bone loss and rebuild your bone core? We address these questions and more as we take you on the journey to creating new or better pathways to bone health.

Women are particularly at higher risk of bone loss because they tend to have smaller, thinner bones than men. Estrogen decreases sharply when you transition through menopause, which results in bone loss. So, the chance of developing bone loss increases as you reach menopause. And in the years after menopause, your body's ability to make new bone can't keep up replacing the bone that has been lost. This is one reason why some women choose to be on estrogen therapy in their post-menopausal years as a protective mechanism for their bone health.

TESTING FOR BONE HEALTH

You can find out if you have already lost bone and are at greater risk of a fracture before it gets to that point. The first step, a bone mineral density (BMD) test, provides a snapshot of your bone health. The most widely recognized BMD test is called a dual-energy x-ray absorptiometry (DXA, also called DEXA) test. A DXA test uses x-rays to measure bone density at your hip and spine. Then your BMD results are compared with those of healthy young adults (your T-score) and age-matched adults (your Z-score).

DOI: 10.1201/9781003250968-12

WHAT DOES MY T-SCORE MEAN?

- A T-score between +1 and −1 is considered normal or healthy.
- A T-score between −1 and −2.5 indicates low bone density, or osteopenia. Bone density is lower than normal but not low enough to be considered osteoporosis.
- A T-score of −2.5 or lower indicates osteoporosis, or excessive bone loss, in which the density and quality of bones are reduced. The greater the negative number, the more severe the osteoporosis. For example, a T-score of −4.0 indicates more severe osteoporosis than a T-score of −3.5.

After you have your T-score, the next step is to determine your FRAX score, which estimates the probability of a fracture within the next 10 years (by use of a web-based calculator tool). The higher the FRAX score, the greater the risk of fracture. The FRAX score helps guide treatment decisions, specifically if medication is indicated.

Professional societies and the U.S. Preventive Services Task Force universally recommend routine osteoporosis screening with BMD testing for women 65 and older. Consider screening earlier than age 65 if you have any risk factors such as low body weight, parental history of hip fracture, and/or a smoking history. However, Medicare doesn't typically start covering the cost of screening DXA tests until age 65, so you may need to advocate for earlier screening if you have risk factors.

CLINICAL PERSPECTIVES

Many postmenopausal women in Carolyn's practice often voiced concerns about their bone health, wanting to learn about integrative approaches that could help them optimize their lifestyle and avoid medication. A diagnosis of osteoporosis or significant bone loss comes with a recommendation to start medication to reduce the risk of a future fracture. Yet it is estimated that as many as 90% of women do not start taking the drug! Why? The biggest reason is that most women are very concerned about potential side effects and are skeptical about the benefits versus the risks of being on long-term medication. There is a growing mistrust of expert medical advice and the pharmaceutical industry when it comes to drugs for osteoporosis.

The osteoporosis drugs in question are typically bisphosphonates. Even though side effects such as osteonecrosis (bone death) of the jaw or atypical fractures near the top of the femur (thigh bone) are rare, the possibility strikes terror in many women. The idea of taking a drug for a year or longer to reduce the risk—of something that may never happen—can be a tough sell. Most women are far more disturbed by the perception of risk than by the probability of harm. So, instead, they prefer to make changes in their lifestyle that can help reduce the risk of bone loss and avoid medication. This can be a reasonable approach if a woman commits to the appropriate changes in her lifestyle and if her bone density remains stable.

Beth, now age 67, had a T-score of −2.2 in her left hip. Two years prior, her T-score has been −1.9, so her newest DXA test result was showing significant low bone density as well as ongoing bone loss. She had not followed the previous advice of her endocrinologist to start on osteoporosis medication (Fosamax). During our conversation, Beth admitted that she did not exercise regularly, although she was active with shopping and housework. She thought she ate reasonably well and took vitamin D most days, but she didn't know if her calcium intake met the recommended amount of 1,200 mg per day. When I raised the possibility of taking Fosamax, Beth was adamant about not taking medication because a friend of hers had done so and had fractured her leg.

Beth was also somewhat resistant to changing her lifestyle, but as we discussed options, she agreed to start a weight-bearing walking program of 10,000 steps a day, take a daily calcium supplement, and see a physical therapist to help build her core strength. After a year of these changes, she would have another DXA test. She agreed that if her T-score then moved into the osteoporosis range, she would be open to taking medication. However, if her T-score was then stable, she would continue with the lifestyle changes and calcium supplement and repeat the DXA in 2 years.

It is certainly frustrating to do all the right things, adjusting your lifestyle to optimize your health, and yet still have progressive bone loss. Osteoporosis has a strong genetic component, so do not blame yourself for factors you cannot control. Given that the consequences of osteoporotic fractures can be serious, medication may be worth considering. As an example, hip fractures cause up to a 25% increase in mortality within 1 year of the incident, and up to 25% of women require long-term care after a hip fracture.[3] A woman who has osteoporosis (especially is she has had a previous fracture) needs to consult with a pharmacist or an endocrinologist about medication options. Making a reasonable choice involves a careful review of the risks and benefits of medication and shared decision-making.[4]

OSTEOPOROSIS MEDICATIONS

Understanding how osteoporosis medications work may be helpful. The cells of your bones are constantly being both lost and built. The cells that remove old or damaged bone are called osteoclasts, while the cells that build new bone are called osteoblasts.

Osteoporosis Medications

Drug Type	How It Works	Examples with Generic (Trade) Names

Antiresorptive drugs	Slow bone breakdown
	Maintain and improve bone mass
		Bisphosphonates
		  Alendronate (Fosamax) oral, and others
		  Zoledronic acid (Zometa, Reclast) IV
		Denosumab (Prolia)

Anabolic drugs	Increase bone formation	Teriparatide (Forteo) Abaloparatide (Tymlos)
Estrogen	Stimulates bone building Slows bone breakdown	Estrogen products Raloxifene (Evista)

So, it makes sense that osteoporosis medications are aimed at decreasing the activity of osteoclasts or increasing the activity of osteoblasts.

MUSCLE HEALTH AND SARCOPENIA

Muscle health is central to bone health because strong muscles help to support the bones. The term *sarcopenia* refers to loss of skeletal muscle mass. It is one of the most influential causes of functional decline and loss of independence in older women.

Many women do not realize that there are ways to slow or possibly even reverse this condition. It does not have to be an inevitable decline. Although a decline in physical activity is one reason that sarcopenia happens, other contributing factors include hormonal changes, chronic illness, inflammation, and poor nutrition. Eating adequate protein (discussed in Chapter 9) to enhance muscle mass requires at least 0.54 grams of protein per pound of ideal body weight (normal BMI). You might add a consultation with a physical therapist to your wellness web to help prevent bone fracture and support your overall bone and muscle health.

BRIDGING THE GAP

In conventional medicine, bone health is on the checklist of healthcare guidelines for postmenopausal women. This typically requires a DXA test, which is generally advised at age 65. If osteoporosis is found or the FRAX score is high (>3), then practitioners often advise starting medication. The rub comes when many women want to know more about what all this means and little information is provided, other than "here's a prescription." Women are often fearful about these medications, and the issue gets lost in the complexity of other health concerns.

This is the time for self-advocacy. Ask for an explanation of your DXA score and your options for treatment. It's important that your provider helps you understand the pros and cons of medication and what else you can do to support your bone health. If your provider can't provide that information to you in an understandable way, then you need to find someone who can.

INTEGRATIVE STRATEGIES

Integrative strategies for bone health in postmenopausal women focus on prevention and management. Successful prevention strategies depend on your knowledge and self-efficacy, which work together to help you modify your behavior and develop healthy habits. First, you need to address factors that contribute to a higher risk of developing bone loss, osteoporosis, and fracture risk. Cigarette smoking, lack of exercise, and insufficient intake of calcium or vitamin D are well-known contributors, and these factors must be considered in the years before menopause. The sooner in life you address these factors, the better off your bones will be as you get older. Other factors, such as genetics and loss of estrogen through menopause, are largely out of your control. Do keep in mind that you can adjust and manage with lifestyle strategies to preserve and strengthen your bones no matter your age.

Nourishment

Food as Medicine

Numerous nutrients are key when it comes to building and maintaining bone strength. The obvious nutrient is calcium. Either from dietary sources or a supplement, calcium has been shown to decrease bone loss in postmenopausal women. The recommended dietary allowance for adults older than 51 is 1,200 mg per day. Foods that are high in calcium include broccoli, kale, collard greens, mustard greens, squash, beans, and legumes.

The dairy industry promotes milk as the best source of calcium, but approximately 65% of the population has a reduced ability to digest lactose, which is the sugar that is found in milk. Other scientific studies about milk and osteoporosis contradict the conventional wisdom that dairy consumption helps reduce osteoporotic fractures. For example, a 12-year-long Nurses' Health Study found that those who consumed the most calcium from dairy foods broke more bones than those who drank less milk.[5] The point is that many factors contribute to how calcium is absorbed and what kind of calcium is best for bones. Consuming calcium through dietary sources is currently the safest way for you to meet the recommended calcium intake. If you are unable to consume adequate calcium through diet alone, then supplementation is needed. If you do not know if you are getting enough calcium in your diet, keep a diary of your food intake for a typical day, and add up the milligrams of calcium consumed. If the total is more than 1,000 mg, you are likely getting enough calcium and don't need a supplement. If the total is less than 1,000 mg, add a calcium citrate supplement at 500 mg daily. Also, be aware that more is not necessarily better. For example, too much calcium supplementation has been associated with an increased risk of heart attacks. Not all calcium supplements are the same, so again, this shows the value of working with a functional medicine practitioner to decide what is ideal for you.

Calcium Supplements: The two primary forms of calcium used in supplements are calcium citrate and calcium carbonate. Because calcium carbonate requires stomach acid for absorption, it's best to take this product with food. Calcium citrate

Calcium-Rich Foods

Food	Calcium (mg)
Yogurt, nonfat, 6 oz	187
Cottage cheese 1%, 1 cup	138
Milk, 8 oz	300
Tofu, ½ cup	200
Dark leafy greens (eg, spinach, kale), 1 cup	100
Fortified orange juice, 4 oz	175
Oatmeal, cooked, 1 cup	185
Figs, dried (two)	65
Broccoli, cooked, 1 cup	60

supplements are absorbed more easily than calcium carbonate. They can be taken on an empty stomach and are more readily absorbed by people who are taking acid-reducing medications for heartburn.

Calcium can also be taken as hydroxyapatite, or microcrystalline hydroxyapatite concentrate, which is a bioavailable source of calcium derived from whole bone. Hydroxyapatite also contains other minerals that are naturally found in healthy bone along with the other active and supportive constituents of bone.

Bone Broth: Our grandparents made soups and stews from the bones, cartilage, and connective tissue of animals for nourishment. Now, our meat is deboned for our convenience, and we're missing out on accessible nutrients. Bone broth contains collagen, protein, essential minerals (calcium and magnesium), and amino acids. It has been around since, arguably, our caveman days, making it a true Paleo food. Naturopaths have used bone broth to support bone and joint health as well as digestive health for decades. Consider using bone broth in cooking as a way to provide additional minerals in your diet.

Prevention of Calcium Loss

Can lifestyle behaviors help you avoid losing calcium from your bones? As discussed in Chapter 9, postmenopausal women require adequate protein, but their intake is often lower than what their bodies need. Different sources of dietary protein may have different effects on your bone metabolism. A current debate about the benefits of protein for bone health concerns whether the source of the protein is animal or plant.

Protein: Animal foods provide predominantly acid precursors, whereas protein in vegetable foods provide base precursors not found in animal foods. Over time, excess dietary acid precursors can lead to an accumulation of acid load that may have adverse consequences for your bones. There is some evidence that a high ratio of dietary animal protein to vegetable protein increases bone loss and risk of fracture in postmenopausal women. A high-protein diet, along with adequate calcium and fruits and vegetables, is important for bone health and osteoporosis prevention. Having a balance of plant to animal protein in your diet is so integral to healthful eating and is especially important for your bones and muscles.

Salt: Excessive salt (ie, sodium) intake is associated with increased calcium loss via the kidneys. For postmenopausal women, decreasing sodium intake from 3.4 grams per day (the U.S. average) to less than 2 grams per day can improve skeletal health. Grains, vegetables, fruits, and beans are very low in sodium, unless salt is added to them. Snack foods, canned foods, dairy products, and meat tend to drive up the amount of sodium in the diet.

Caffeine: Whether it comes in coffee or colas, caffeine is a weak diuretic that causes calcium loss via the kidneys. Caffeine intakes of more than 300 mg per day have been shown to accelerate bone loss in older postmenopausal women. However, one to two cups of coffee a day are not harmful.

Tobacco: Long-term smokers have 10% weaker bones and a 40% higher risk of fractures as they age. Even secondhand smoke can negatively affect bone density.

Medications: Common medications, including proton-pump inhibitors taken for heartburn (eg, Prilosec, Prevacid), glucocorticoids (such as prednisone), aromatase

Magnesium-Rich Foods

Food	Serving Size	Amount of Magnesium (mg)
Pumpkin seed, kernels	1 oz	168
Almonds, dry roasted	1 oz	80
Spinach, boiled	½ cup	78
Cashews, dry roasted	1 oz	74
Peanuts, oil roasted	¼ cup	63
Soymilk, plain or vanilla	1 cup	61
Black beans, cooked	½ cup	60
Edamame, shelled, cooked	½ cup	50

inhibitors (used in treatment of some types of breast cancers), some diuretics (eg, Lasix), and some anticonvulsants, have been shown to diminish bone density because they affect how calcium is absorbed and metabolized. If possible, avoiding long-term use is the best medicine.

Supplements

Calcium transport in the body occurs at three primary sites: intestines, bone, and kidney. Equilibrium is maintained by the interplay of calcium absorbed from the intestines, movement of calcium into and out of the bones, and the kidney's recovery and excretion of calcium into the urine. Both vitamin D and vitamin K play a role in maintaining this delicate balance.

Vitamin D is essential for growth and maintenance of healthy bones throughout life. It is absorbed from the diet or is synthesized in the skin with exposure to sunlight. That is why vitamin D deficiency can be seen in women who live in the northern latitudes, use sunblock, have darker skin pigmentation, work indoors, or wear burkas or other full-body coverings. Food sources of vitamin D include cod liver oil, liver, cheese, egg yolks, and fortified milk. It is hard to get enough vitamin D from food, and given warnings about harmful exposure to the sun, it is even more likely that you will need a supplement to maintain healthy vitamin D levels.

As mentioned in Chapter 4, taking a minimum of 1,000 IU vitamin D daily is often needed to maintain a healthy level. The normal range of a vitamin D level is 20–80 ng/mL, so over 40 ng/mL is ideal for maximum health benefits. 25-hydroxy vitamin D, abbreviated 25(OH)D, is the best marker of vitamin D status, and low levels (<30 ng/mL) are associated with a higher risk of hip fracture.

Vitamin K is another essential vitamin for bone formation. Your body uses vitamin K to produce osteocalcin, a protein found in large amounts in bone. Epidemiological studies suggest that a diet with high levels of vitamin K is associated with a lower risk of hip fractures in older women. There are two forms of vitamin K (vitamin K_1 and vitamin K_2), which come from different sources and have different biological activity. Vitamin K_1, the predominant source of vitamin K in the diet, is found in high concentrations in green leafy vegetables and certain vegetable oils and is present in lower concentrations in meat, milk, cheese, eggs, and fermented soybeans (natto). MK4 and MK7 are two types of vitamin K_2 that are commercially available in dietary supplements.

Magnesium works together with calcium to relax muscles and move fluids through cells for optimal bone health. Magnesium is a cofactor for alkaline phosphatase, an enzyme involved in bone mineralization. Adequate intake of magnesium is essential in postmenopausal women. The optimal ratio of calcium to magnesium for bone health is 2 to 1, with a daily ideal for women of 1,000 mg of calcium and 500 mg of magnesium. Many foods contain magnesium (see also Chapter 4 for various formulations of magnesium supplements).

Other nutrients needed for bone health include boron, manganese, zinc, strontium, and DHEA. These nutrients can be obtained from a nutrient-dense diet and can be supplemented in a quality bone health formula.

We recommend that you consult a functional medicine practitioner or naturopath to discuss the supplements that are best for you. At a minimum, make sure that every day you take 1,000 IU of vitamin D, 500 mg of calcium and 250 mg magnesium. Also make sure to eat the recommended amounts of green leafy vegetables.

Exercise and Movement

Any exercise is better than none, and some activities are especially good for bone health. When it comes to building bone and slowing bone loss, you need weight-bearing exercises that force your body to work against gravity, such as walking, climbing stairs, jogging, or playing tennis or similar activities. However, *to strengthen bone* you also need exercises in which you move against some kind of resistance, such as lifting weights. Exercises that use your own body weight as resistance, such as push-ups and planks, are also great options. Strengthening the muscles around the bones is also important. For instance, strengthening your back muscles can reduce your risk of vertebral fractures (which leads to that hunched, stooping posture you see in many older women). Strengthening your core muscles will help with balance, stability, and effective joint movement.

Muscle mass naturally diminishes with age, but regular strength training and eating adequate protein can help you preserve and enhance your muscles. Building lean muscle mass will also help you lose weight and control your body fat, because lean muscle mass burns calories more efficiently. Sound good?

As you venture into your later years, remaining physically active is crucial to enjoying life and remaining in your best health. Understanding and then lowering the risk of osteoporosis can ensure bone health is maintained and support the process of successfully aging. A sedentary lifestyle and low physical activity are risk factors for osteoporotic bone fractures, as well as many other health conditions. You should aim for at least 30 minutes of physical activity that includes weight-bearing on most days (preferably daily) and at least 2 days per week of muscle-strengthening activities.

Qigong and *Tai Chi* are both ancient Chinese traditions that involve a series of slow, graceful body movements with deep breathing. They are known for their ability to improve balance, coordination, and muscle strength, and to reduce the risk of falls. These practices were developed as meditative movements rather than to increase heart rates or burn calories. Because they are low impact and put minimal stress on muscles and joints, they are safe for all ages and fitness levels.

Qigong combines mental concentration, breathing techniques, and body movements to activate and cultivate "vital energy." In Chinese philosophy, *qi* or *chi* (pronounced "chee") means air or breath, and *gong* means work or cultivation; when combined, they are translated to mean "the art of cultivating vital energy." Qigong roots go back thousands of years and stem from the practice of cultivating qi primarily for health benefits.

Tai Chi has the same basic properties (qi), fundamental principle (relaxation), and fundamental method (slowness) but was developed later as a martial art. However, after being introduced into the West, it has been modified for various health benefit and health conditions. For example, patients with mild-to-moderate Parkinson disease benefit from Tai Chi training because it reduces balance impairments, which, in turn, improves functional capacity and decreases falls.

Chi walking blends the health benefits of walking with the core principles of Tai Chi to deliver maximum physical, mental, and spiritual fitness. Becoming a better walker does not depend on how fast or how far you can walk but on how well you can listen to your body and respond to its needs. Chi walking can be ideal for women as they age because it encourages good body mechanics, improves balance, and engages the core. A quick explanation:

> *Begin by aligning your posture, making sure your spine is long, tall, and straight. Set your feet hip-width apart and parallel and soften your knees. Then, engage your core by leveling your pelvis. Do this by placing a hand on your belly with your thumb at your naval and your fingers just above your pubic bone, and gently activating the pelvic muscles under your fingers so that your pelvis tilts. Your body weight is always centered over your leading foot, so that movement begins from your center, and the bulk of the work is done by your core muscles rather than your feet and legs. This enhances balance and lessens the risk of falling or injury. Next, move forward by leading with your upper body, in balance over your stepping foot, rather than leading with your legs. Choose which direction you are going before you start, so that all parts are moving in the same direction. Keep moving forward, with your posture straight, your core engaged, and your upper body balanced over your lower body. Mindfully complete the first four steps so that your forward movement has balance, purpose, and direction. Watching a YouTube video is helpful to see this in action.*

Nordic walking is a type of total body walking done with walking poles that are similar to ski poles. It has been done in Scandinavian countries for years, and now an estimated 12 million Europeans are Nordic walkers. This full-body workout helps to engage the core and upper-body muscles, which in turn support posture and stability. Getting into a walking rhythm can increase the exertion of walking by 40%, as well as being a form of moving meditation. Nordic walking can be done even in winter months, by yourself or in a group as a social activity—what a fun way to benefit from a daily walking routine.

Healing Systems

Yoga

In addition to the form and benefits of yoga discussed in Chapters 4 and 6, yoga also benefits bone health. Yoga is a safe and gentle way to encourage mobility for the spine and provide benefits for both bones and balance. In *Yoga for Osteoporosis*, yoga therapist Ellen Saltonstall and Dr. Loren Fishman provide an excellent demonstration of safe poses for women with osteopenia and osteoporosis.[6]

For women of any age, weight-bearing yoga postures that move the body against resistance, like table pose and plank pose, strengthen bones and increase endurance. Balance postures, like the tree pose, reduce risk of falling. To counter a tendency toward age-related rounding of the upper spine, doing back-strengthening postures such as baby cobra (with arms at the sides) and the locust pose are beneficial. Some versions may need to be modified, but make sure you are still doing the poses correctly. Proper alignment in poses maximizes your bone's ability to resist any applied force, so you need good instruction and constant attention to reducing the risk of injury. Seek out an instructor who focuses on good form and correct alignment of the pose and encourages the use of blocks and cushions for support.

The episode in television's *Grace and Frankie*, when Jane Fonda can't get herself up off the toilet, reminded Carolyn of her recent struggle getting up from the floor after playing with her grandboys.

> *Because I have osteopenia (T-score 1.9), I wanted to get expert advice so that I didn't injure myself while exercising. I sought help from a physical therapist also trained in yoga. She gave me specific poses to strengthen my weak gluteal (butt) muscles and boost my core muscle endurance, both of which are needed to get up from the floor. I knew that the plank position is valuable for these muscle groups, but I have always found it difficult and avoided it. Ironically, this was the first exercise my physical therapist wanted me to do. Why? Quite simply, the plank is a bodyweight exercise that boosts core muscle endurance and improves the glutes.*

Muscle *endurance* refers to the ability of a muscle to hold a sustained contraction for a longer period of time. This means you can continue using your muscles over and over before they fatigue (such as while walking, running, or repeating an exercise several times). Muscle *strength* refers to the amount of force a muscle can exert or how much weight you can lift. Strength is what gives you the power to exert a maximal force (such as lifting a heavy box). When it comes to your core muscles, improving your endurance can help you maintain posture, support your spine, and keep you aligned while you are sitting, standing, and walking. (And yes, helps you get up more easily from the floor or off the toilet seat!)

Planks build your core by working both your abdominal wall muscles and your glutes. While doing a plank, make sure you consciously focus on tightening your glutes to avoid depending solely on your abdominal muscles. Gradually build up to being able to hold a plank pose for between 1 and 2 minutes. This is roughly how long most exercise sets last, and you want your core to at least be strong enough to maintain your spine in a neutral position for this amount of time.

Yoga offers many options. There are various types of yoga practices to fit your needs, and standard poses can be modified if needed. For example, chair yoga is a great option for if you have balance, flexibility, or other physical concerns.

Postural Restoration and Alignment

As you age, your body posture and alignment also change due to loss of bone mass and muscle integrity. Have you ever seen your reflection and noticed that your head is leading the way, or your shoulders and upper back are rounded forward? This stooped, slouched posture is often associated with older women. The good news is that you can intentionally retrain your postural alignment. Practicing good body alignment and correcting body positions that create imbalance can help you avoid falls and fractures as well as help with your proprioception, which is the body's ability to sense where it is in space. Examples include knowing whether your feet are on grass or cement, being able to balance on one leg, and touching your nose with your finger with your eyes closed. In other words, good proprioception is essential for your body to move normally and maintain balance. Unfortunately, proprioception declines with age, impairing balance and increasing the chances of falling.

Postural alignment therapies use gentle corrective exercises to restore alignment and balance. The focus is on correction of underlying dysfunction, rather than treating symptoms. These therapies include reeducating your body to address injuries and improve coordination and habitual patterns of movement that have become inefficient. Fortunately, pathways in your neuromuscular system have *plasticity,* which means they can be modified in response not just to injury but also to training. You may want to check for practitioners in your community who offer one of the following methods of practice.

The *Alexander Technique* is a body alignment program to reduce tension in the head, neck, and back, named after its developer, Frederick Matthias Alexander (1869–1955). His techniques improve posture and movement, especially those caused by poor habits—which can be easy to fall into. The Alexander Technique teaches you to be more aware of your body and how to improve poor posture and move more efficiently. A typical lesson involves taking a close look at your patterns during common movements (eg, bending, walking, reaching, sitting at the computer, standing). Being aware of how you move and hold tension in your body helps to retrain and realign your body so that everyday actions can reduce muscle tension and improve posture.

The *Feldenkrais Method* is named after its originator, Dr. Moshé Feldenkrais (1904–1984), who drew from several sources, including the Alexander Technique, martial arts, psychology, and biomechanics. This method uses two formats: group work for movement sequences and individual work for manipulation. The Feldenkrais Method involves a process of organic learning, movement, and sensing to free you from habitual patterns and allow for new patterns of thinking, moving, and feeling to emerge. Posture, coordination, and flexibility are improved through reprogramming your neuromuscular system to sense more accurately and be more aware of muscular effort.

Catherine was treated for several years by a Feldendkrais practitioner for chronic back pain.

My Feldenkrais teacher had me relearn some basics: how to walk, how to sit and stand from a chair, how to ride my bike, and even how to move the muscles in my belly and face. Feldenkrais involves listening to my body and learning how it feels when it is well aligned. Paying attention to and heightening awareness of how my body moves helped reduce the pain and improve my posture and balance.

Feldenkrais explores the biological and cultural aspects of movement, posture, and learning. It enables you to see how your habits can limit you to a small portion of your potential. Each of us has a personal history—our upbringing, culture, injuries, illnesses—through which we have developed our own patterns of physical and psychological behavior and responses. These patterns are deeply embedded in our nervous system, and over time can become dysfunctional, creating unnecessary physical and psychological limitations.

Rolfing is a bodywork technique that involves deep manipulation of the fascia and soft tissue to improve body alignment and balance. Rolfing was named after its creator, Dr. Ida Rolf (1896–1979), who more than 50 years ago recognized that the body is a system of networks of tissue rather than a collection of separate parts. The Rolfing process enables the body to regain the natural integrity of its form, thus enhancing muscular and postural efficiency and freedom of movement. It has also been shown to significantly reduce chronic stress and reduce spinal curvature in individuals with swayback (lordosis). However, because Rolfing is a deep-tissue approach and usually involves a series of treatments, it may be painful for women who are sensitive to pressure.

———

Flexibility, agility, and good posture and body alignment are all essential to good bone health. Consider including in your wellness web of healers a practitioner who focuses on postural restoration. Find a yoga class that meets your particular needs. You might even take dance lessons! Any or all of these approaches will keep you moving and create new pathways to build the core. Remember, unlike many conditions, bones are silent until something goes wrong.

PATHWAYS TO BUILD YOUR CORE

Self-Awareness: What prompted you to start thinking about your bones? Do you have any risk factors that warrant early screening?

Self-Compassion: Listen to your own wants and needs as you navigate the options for healthy bones. Trust yourself to make the choices that are best for you.

Self-Advocacy: What preventive strategies are you engaged in for bone health? If you have bone issues, what management interventions are you willing to consider to build your core?

———

Catherine's Pathway

I became aware of bone health, or a lack thereof, at an early age because of my mother. Now age 96, she has had two hip replacements (the first at age 55), two major hip repairs, one knee replacement, and two major back surgeries. None of these were due to falls, so I imagine heredity is involved. However, starting in her early 30s through her early 90s, my mother broke many bones (femur, collarbone, both ankles, and wrist) that were due to falls. She also shattered her pelvis and another femur. In sum, my mother has been in bone-related pain for over 60 years. Thus far, I have been able to avoid any broken bones or joint replacements. However, many of my health-conscious friends are falling and breaking—wrists, shoulders, arms, ribs, femurs, ankles. I am reminded that we are not immune to breaking bones. I'm embarrassed to admit that it has been 7 years since my last DXA scan. It seems like I've become complacent about monitoring my bone health, perhaps assuming that good news 7 years ago still holds. I wonder.

For the past 40+ years, I have turned to alternative health practitioners to improve back pain and support bone health. I started with biofeedback, Alexander Technique, and yoga. Once I moved to Chicago, I worked for many years with a doctor of naprapathy, followed by work with a Feldenkrais master, and most recently, a Chinese-trained acupuncturist. Since 2007, the constant has been my personal trainer who combines multiple modalities for core and muscle strength along with balance. With encouragement from my physical therapist, I purchased a recumbent stationary bike for seniors and actually like using it, regularly.

The next step is to have a DXA scan to see how my bones are doing and whether additional interventions are suggested. I am not keen on taking more medications but, if needed, want to be properly informed. This might not be about bones per se, but I finally acknowledged that my mattress, sofa, and even my car were the causes of considerable pain. Within a span of 6 months, I made all new purchases, and my core and bones feel much happier.

11 Brain Health
Stimulate New Pathways

"Where did I put my keys?" "I know her, but what is her name?" "Who was the lead actor in that movie we watched the other night?" Joan Lunden wrote a popular book about this phenomenon: *Why Did I Come into This Room?*[1] These are the daily questions that cause us to wonder: Am I losing my memory? Could these be signs of early dementia?

When you hear the words *brain health*, what first comes to mind? Do you wonder about the qualities of a healthy brain? Or whether there is a way to avoid dementia? The news media and advertising belabor the brain's vulnerability to decline with age. Difficulties with memory, language, and logical thinking are typically associated with some form of dementia. However, other conditions might be the cause, such as depression, vitamin deficiency, thyroid disorders, vision loss, hearing impairment, and some medications—and some of these can be managed or are even reversible. In any case, anyone showing these signs should have a thorough medical evaluation.

Nonetheless, dementia has become a widespread condition among aging adults in the United States. You may have had a parent, grandparent, partner, or friend who has been affected by dementia. The impact on the individual and family members can be devastating. Because dementia is so feared, we'll examine it first before delving into the healthy brain.

DEMENTIA

Dementia is characterized by a decline in mental abilities, including memory, language, and logical thinking, that is severe enough to affect daily living. There are different types of dementia:

Neurodegenerative dementia, commonly called Alzheimer disease, is caused by loss of brain tissue. It is the most common type of dementia.

Vascular dementia is caused by poor blood flow to the brain. Strokes, heart disease, diabetes, high blood pressure, high cholesterol, all increase the risk of vascular dementia.

Alzheimer disease is the most common cause of dementia. According to the Alzheimer's Association, more than 5 million Americans are affected, a number projected to increase to nearly 14 million by 2050. It is rare in people younger than 60 and likely to be associated with specific genetic mutations.[2] According to Lisa Mosconi, director of the Women's Brain Initiative and author of *The XX Brain*, two out of every three patients with Alzheimer disease are women.[3] A stunning fact is

DOI: 10.1201/9781003250968-13

that women in their 60s are twice as likely to develop Alzheimer disease than they are to develop breast cancer. Yet, breast cancer has far greater visibility than Alzheimer disease, so much so that brain health of the aging woman is often overlooked.

The onset of Alzheimer disease is insidious. Episodic memory decreases, with poor recall of recent events, slowed speech, and inability to remember names. These negative changes are the result of various genetic, medical, and lifestyle factors. Some experts claim that Alzheimer disease actually begins to develop silently in the brain 20–30 years before the first symptoms appear. Recent estimates suggest that more than 46 million Americans are now affected by this initial, or preclinical, stage of the disease.

Lois, age 71, was concerned about her short-term memory loss. Over the last year, she noticed difficulty with finding words, getting confused with directions when driving, forgetting appointments, and repeating herself. She had recently become anxious about giving business presentations, fearful she might forget words, repeat herself, or simply become confused while speaking. She wanted testing to establish a baseline and determine what objective findings for memory loss could be identified. Her father had developed Alzheimer disease in his 70s, and she feared the same diagnosis. Lois's neuropsych testing showed mild cognitive impairment, MCI, which, although unsettling news, confirmed her suspicion that something was wrong.

MILD COGNITIVE IMPAIRMENT

MCI can be diagnosed with formal cognitive testing. It refers to the stage between the expected cognitive decline of normal aging and the more serious decline of dementia. In MCI, like in other forms of cognitive impairment, difficulties with memory, language, thinking, and judgment are greater than the changes normally expected with age. If you have MCI, you may be aware that your memory or mental function has "slipped." Your family and close friends also may notice a change. But, in general, these changes won't significantly interfere with your daily life and usual activities, such as driving, managing medications, and cooking. Nonetheless, MCI may increase the risk of developing dementia or Alzheimer disease in the future.

Aging women may identify with Lois and wonder what to do to stop the condition from progressing. Before we delve into how to treat Lois with her MCI, let's look at contributing factors that play a role in dementia.

CONTRIBUTING FACTORS

Genetics: Although genes can play a role in a small percentage of the population, in general, genes are not your destiny. As an example, *APOE4* is a gene variant that increases your risk of Alzheimer disease but does not actually cause it. In fact, more than 60% of patients with Alzheimer disease do not carry *APOE4*. Scientists believe that the vast majority of cases of Alzheimer disease are caused by a complex combination of genetic and nongenetic determinants. Research is ongoing to disentangle these genetic constellations.

APOE4

APOE4 is a genetic marker for Alzheimer disease. Carrying one *APOE4* gene (inherited from one parent) increases your lifetime risk of Alzheimer disease to 30%. Carrying two *APOE4* genes (one from each parent) increases your lifetime risk to greater than 50%.

Epigenetics is the study of how your behaviors and environment can cause changes in how your genes work. Unlike genetic changes, epigenetic changes are reversible. Your DNA is not changed, but epigenetic changes can change how your body reads your DNA. This means that by optimizing positive health strategies that you can control—your environment, lifestyle, nutrition, and hormone health—you can influence your brain health. Taking care of your brain is a preventive measure that must begin early in life and continue during your later decades. Recent research on "epigenetic reprogramming" in mice offers distant promise for reversing the aging clock in people. But don't wait around for scientific evidence before making positive lifestyle shifts.

Genomics is the study of a person's complete set of genes, including how those genes interact with each other and with the person's environment. Each of us has about 25,000 different genes made up of approximately 3 billion DNA units. Subtle variations in DNA are what not only make us look different from one another but also create subtle health differences. The knowledge of health risks and benefits gained by understanding your genomic profile may provide a foundation for planning a personalized approach to lifestyle modification. If you are interested in learning about your genomic profile, we encourage you to have a discussion with your functional medicine practitioner. If you decide that this approach may be beneficial, your practitioner can order genomic testing, which can provide direction on how to improve your quality of life, no matter your age.

Nutrition and nutrient deficiencies are becoming increasingly recognized as a significant contributor to brain health. The AARP 2017 Brain Health and Nutrition Survey of adults 40 and older produced notable findings.[4] Most survey respondents simply are not getting proper nutrition. Virtually none of the respondents consumed the USDA-recommended number of servings in all five food groups (fruits and vegetables, starches, dairy, protein, and fat). One-third of respondents did not consume the recommended amount in *any* food group. The good news was that adults who ate at least the recommended amounts of fruits and vegetables reported better brain health and scored above average on mental well-being tests.

BRIDGING THE GAP

If you or a loved one is confronted with memory loss and changes, you'll want to see your physician to determine whether these are signs of early dementia. In addition to learning as much as possible about your health history, your physician will ask you to take some cognitive question-and-answer style tests to get a reading of your reasoning, orientation, and attention skills. Often, neurological testing is done to evaluate your language, memory, movement, and balance skills. Blood tests and advanced brain-imaging tests may also help identify whether your symptoms are being caused by other health conditions. Even with testing, early diagnoses of conditions like Alzheimer disease and related disorders can be challenging because the loss of skills and function may be subtle. There is yet no single behavioral marker that can reliably discriminate Alzheimer disease from the other dementias.

Despite robust and well-funded research, no drug treatment has been found to cure Alzheimer disease. Clinical trials on various drugs have had disappointing results. The currently available drugs (eg, donepezil, rivastigmine, memantine) address only symptoms and are of limited efficacy. Plus, response to medication varies for each person and may not work for everyone. However, these drugs may slow the progression of the Alzheimer disease and make it easier to live with. Research continues to look for novel drug approaches to manage the disease. In the meantime, you need to do whatever you can to support good brain health.

INTEGRATIVE STRATEGIES

Over the last 100 years, Western science led us to believe that after adolescence, the brain was fixed. It would not change again until aging triggered the long process of decline, and brain cells could not be replaced. New science tells us otherwise. In *The Brain That Changes Itself*, Dr. Norman Doidge describes neuroplasticity as the brain's ability to adapt, change, and restructure physiologically.[5] Neuro stands for neurons, which are the nerve cells in your brain, and plastic means changeable, malleable, or modifiable. So, what does this mean on a practical basis? It means that your brain is not static; it can develop new neural pathways and connections. Neurosurgeon Dr. Sanjay Gupta reminds us in *Keep Sharp*, "to constantly be using new paths and trails and roads within our brain. No matter how old you are, it's never too late to develop new brain pathways."[6]

REWIRING NEW BRAIN PATHWAYS

How can you create new pathways in your brain? Dr. Gupta wisely asserts that trying something new can connect new pathways to improve and maintain memory. Learn a new language, take up painting, become a blogger, or return to the piano lessons you abandoned years ago. One of Carolyn's friends started ukulele lessons when she was 60 and is strumming away in a ukulele club. Similarly, podcast guest Zib Hinz (episode #81) learned to play cello at age 65 and now performs in a chamber group. Anything outside your normal patterns will harness other areas of the brain.

Many of the women featured on the podcast *Women Over 70: Aging Reimagined* engage in activities that stimulate their brains and result in enjoyment and accomplishment. For example, when 83-year-old Recille Hamrel's (episode #20) storytelling venue was disrupted by the pandemic, she learned how to paint with watercolors and, in less than 2 years, exhibited her work. At age 87, Karla Klinger (episode #4) selected poems she had written over the decades for her first book-length publication, *Life Unfolding*. For her 100th birthday, fun-loving Marion Giles (episode #58) threw a cocktail party for 100 people and a llama, a parrot, and a monkey from the Brookfield Zoo. Might now be a good time to reignite your passion for a former hobby or start a new one?

BRAIN HEALTH

Brain health is the preservation of optimal brain integrity and mental and cognitive function at a given age in the absence of overt brain diseases that affect normal brain function.[7-8]

Let's now shift attention from a disease model of the brain to qualities of a healthy aging brain. Dr. Laura Baker, at the 2021 Dementia Prevention Conference, reported that studies of exercise, cognitive and social stimulation, and diet show that each of these factors can reduce the risk of dementia.[7] A combination of all may have a more powerful and synergistic effect. These are the results of a large, long-term randomized controlled trial demonstrating that a multidomain lifestyle intervention can improve cognitive function in older adults from the general population who are at increased risk of developing dementia.[8] The work of Dr. Richard Isaacson, a neurologist and founder of the Alzheimer's Prevention Clinic at Weill Cornell Medicine and New York-Presbyterian, supports Dr. Baker's findings on brain health. He reinforces the concept that cognition should be considered as an everyday essential, at any age and throughout the life span.

NOURISHMENT

Sleep: This critical piece of brain health is one of the pillars of health (described in detail in Chapter 6). We have all experienced that we do not think well when we are tired. Our brain cannot function well without adequate sleep. This is another important reminder that good sleep quality is a non-negotiable ingredient for memory, learning, and proper functioning. A good night's sleep also detoxifies the brain by clearing debris and metabolic waste. In *XX Brain*, Dr. Lisa Mosconi points out that both too little sleep and fragmented sleep have been linked to increased accumulation of the brain plaques found in Alzheimer disease.[3]

Estrogen: In Chapter 4, we covered the use of estrogen therapy in considerable detail. After menopause, your brain changes and needs to find new ways to perform efficiently. Hormones play many functions: in addition to keeping your brain energized, hormones keep your bones, gut, immune function, and sex life strong. Despite these many benefits, keep in mind that estrogen therapy is not appropriate for every woman. The choice to be on hormone therapy for brain health is an important discussion to have with your health provider.

Hydration: Your brain is strongly influenced by hydration status. The brain is 2% of your body weight and receives 20% of your blood circulation at any time—it depends on you being well hydrated. Even mild dehydration, such as the loss of 1%–3% of body weight, can impair brain function. A basic step is keeping water within easy reach. Have a water bottle with you all the time. Start your morning by drinking a glass of water, and drink at least four and up to eight 8-ounce glasses (about a half-gallon or 2 liters) of water every day.

Obesity: Evidence to date suggests that obesity is associated with altered brain structure and reduced cognitive function, neuroplasticity, and brain volume. Particularly in midlife, obesity is associated with mild cognitive impairment and Alzheimer disease. The mechanism by which obesity influences cognitive function is not well understood, but it appears that extra weight is not good for brain health.

Food as Medicine

Diet mediates risk of dementia through indirect yet very effective pathways. Diets rich in vegetables, berries, nuts, fish, lean proteins, and healthy fats improve virtually all metabolic processes. This in turn reduces the risk of cerebrovascular disease, which is a driver of vascular dementia and a risk factor for Alzheimer disease.

One of few studies currently available on diet and the brain is the MIND diet study, which is a combination of a Mediterranean–DASH diet intervention for neurodegenerative delay (discussed in Chapter 9). The diet emphasizes natural and plant-based foods with limited intakes of animal-based and high saturated fat foods. Those who strictly adhered to the diet had a 53% reduction in risk for Alzheimer's disease, and those who adhered moderately had a 35% reduction.[9]

Dan Buettner, author of *Blue Zones*, identified places in the world where a high percentage of people enjoy remarkably long lives, some well past 100 years old.[10] When asked what factors improve brain health and longevity, he noted that nutrition is the optimal choice among all lifestyle factors. Buettner's meta-analysis of 154 dietary surveys in five blue zones revealed that 95% of the 100-year-olds ate plant-based diets, including plenty of beans.

Dr. Dale Bredesen, neurologist and author of *The End of Alzheimer's*, advises eating a plant-based diet that is low in starchy carbohydrates and consuming good fats such as olive oil, nuts, and avocados.[11] He also supports intermittent fasting for at least 12 hours between your last meal of the night and your first meal of the next morning. This fast depletes the liver's stores of glycogen and promotes mild ketosis, which can strengthen and protect the brain and nerve cells. Whether or not you choose a fasting program, the bottom line is to reduce your sugar (simple carbohydrate) intake. Although the brain needs glucose (sugar), too much is a bad thing. A diet high in sugar leads to excess glucose in the brain, which has been linked with memory and cognitive deficits. Sugar is best consumed in whole foods that take longer for your body to digest, avoiding the "high-sugar" state.

Supplements

Supplements cannot replace a healthy diet or a healthy lifestyle, so first make sure your diet includes a diversity of foods, with an abundance of foods that are rich in antioxidants. However, even if your diet is excellent, you may need to add a few essential nutrients.

Vitamin D: Along with other reasons to take your vitamin D (at least 1,000–2,000 IU per day) is that it has a major impact on how the brain functions. Emerging evidence shows that vitamin D plays a role in the normal functioning of the central nervous system, including cognition. In 2014, the journal *Neurology* reported findings from a study of over 1,600 participants.[12] Moderate and severe vitamin D deficiency in older adults was associated with more than twice the risk of some forms of dementia, including Alzheimer disease. Studies like this support the need to take your daily dose of vitamin D to maintain a serum level of 40–80 ng/mL.

B complex: If you are under a lot of stress and your diet is not ideal, you might take a B-complex vitamin. Vitamins B_5, B_{12}, and folate, in particular, support your nervous system. With aging, your metabolism naturally slows down, and the absorption of B vitamins, especially B_{12}, may decrease. Some medications, like acid blockers, can also reduce absorption of B vitamins. Certain diets, such as strict vegetarian diets, may lead to a B_{12} deficiency. If you decide to have your levels of B_6, B_{12}, and folate checked, make sure you stop taking any supplements for at least a week before getting your blood drawn.

N-Acetyl-L-Cysteine (NAC): NAC is an amino acid building block for glutathione—one of the most crucial antioxidants in your body, involved in a multitude of metabolic reactions affecting the nervous, immune, and digestive systems. Glutathione is formed from three amino acids: glutamate, glycine, and cysteine. As we age, these amino acids can become depleted and cause oxidative stress (see Chapter 9). That oxidative stress can be reduced by antioxidants, for example, in the form of NAC, which can help your body replenish its stores of glutathione. The recommended dosage of NAC is 600 mg, one to three times a day. We suggest consulting with a functional or integrative medicine practitioner to determine if this supplement is a good choice for you.

Omega-3 and omega-6 fatty acids: These essential fatty acids are not produced in adequate amounts in your body, so they need to be part of your diet. Omega-3 fatty acids help protect your brain cells from the natural wear and tear of aging. Adequate omega-3 levels have been associated with preserved memory, reduced brain shrinkage, and a lower risk of dementia. Two specific omega-3 fatty acids are EPA (eicosapentaenoic acid) and DHA (docosahexaenoic acid). DHA especially has strong anti-inflammatory qualities that are important for brain health.

In contrast to the anti-inflammatory qualities of the omega-3s, certain omega-6 fatty acids such as GLA (gamma-linoleic acid) and ARA (arachidonic acid), are pro-inflammatory. However, despite their pro-inflammatory action, omega-6 fatty acids are still a dietary requirement. What's important is the ratio of omega-3 to omega-6. The root of the problem is that the typical Western diet includes an overabundance of omega-6 fatty acids and getting enough omega-3s is just more difficult. So, you may need to add more omega-3s to your diet, usually in the form of a DHA supplement. Levels of omega-3 and omega-6 fatty acids can be measured by blood tests.

Probiotics and prebiotics: We have said it before—a healthy gut is critical for a healthy brain. You can optimize your gut health by taking probiotics (the right bacteria for your gut) and prebiotics (the right food for those bacteria). In the *Brain*

Maker, Dr. David Perlmutter discusses how healthy gut bacteria help control inflammation, bolster the integrity of the intestinal wall, and produce important chemicals for brain health.[13] An unhealthy gut microbiome can make the microbial population become more inflammatory, producing specialized proteins that induce immune cells to damage neurons in the brain.

Both probiotics and prebiotics are critical to support gut bacteria. Yes, you can take supplements, but dietary sources are, as usual, the best sources. Fermented foods such as kimchi, sauerkraut, sour pickles, miso soup, and kombucha contain live beneficial bacteria and are good probiotics. Yogurt contains probiotics, but it may also contain a lot of sugar. Plus, it's a dairy product, so it may not be your best probiotic unless made at home with known ingredients. Kefir, a fermented milk drink, may be better tolerated. Foods such as jicama, onions, garlic, asparagus, dandelion greens, Jerusalem artichokes, barley, and oats are types of dietary fiber that feed the friendly bacteria in your gut and are good prebiotics.

HEALING SYSTEMS

Evidence is growing that degenerative disorders of the brain are best treated by using a multifactorial approach tailored to individual needs. Various brain health programs and practitioners can evaluate and support improving brain health. One emerging approach is the ReCODE program, developed by Dale Bredesen, MD.

ReCODE

In *The End of Alzheimer's*, Dr. Bredesen promotes the idea that the course of cognitive decline can be altered.[11] His protocol can be useful for individuals with mild cognitive impairment as well as those who already have Alzheimer disease. In addition, those individuals who carry the *APOE4* gene variant that increases risk of Alzheimer disease can take steps to prevent Alzheimer disease or reverse cognitive decline. The evidence for Bredesen's method is in the early stages of research, and further research will likely uncover other gene variants that contribute to the risk of Alzheimer disease.

Using a comprehensive, functional medicine approach, Bredesen reported that cognition improved, both subjectively and objectively, in a small sample of patients. He highlights three processes that contribute to cognitive decline: inflammation, suboptimal nutrients to the brain, and toxic exposures. His program includes ways to activate the innate immune system by reducing inflammation, eliminating toxic substances in the environment (eg, heavy metals like mercury and endocrine-disruption agents like BpA), and engaging in brain activation/retraining with certain computer-based games with cognitive stimulation. The ReCode program is individualized, based on many factors that are identified in a comprehensive evaluation, including blood tests, genetic tests, cognitive assessment, and brain imaging. Anyone interested in pursuing this protocol is advised to read *The End of Alzheimer's* and/or to see an integrative practitioner knowledgeable in Bredesen's principles of brain health.

Exercise

We have been beating the drum about the need for exercise because of its many benefits, so it should not be surprising that exercise also contributes greatly to brain health. Individuals who exercise regularly have slower rates of age-related memory and cognitive decline than those who are more sedentary. Such observations have provided the basis for using exercise to improve memory and cognition in cognitive disorders such as dementia. The following benefits of exercise are good for all of us to keep in mind.

- Exercise increases your body's ability to effectively repair neurons and created new ones. The brain needs oxygen to do its job, and exercise increases delivery of oxygen to all your tissues, including the brain.
- Walking, cycling, or other cardiovascular exercise strengthens the heart and the blood vessels that supply the brain. People who engage in these activities often feel mentally sharper. Don't worry—you don't have to start training to run a marathon or swim the English Channel. Simply walking, at a good pace, stimulates the growth of new neurons. Remember, what you do to keep your heart healthy also keeps your brain healthy.
- Exercise reduces oxidative stress, improves insulin sensitivity, and helps with maintaining normal weight.
- Exercise reduces inflammation and increases clearance of amyloid beta, the main component of the plaques found in the brain in Alzheimer disease.
- Exercise helps to switch on a regenerative protein called brain-derived neurotrophic factor (BDNF) that helps create new and healthy brain cells and increases neuroplasticity.

We can't say it any more plainly: if you want good cognition, your body needs to move. Nothing accelerates brain atrophy more than immobility. As one example, in a small study at the University of Birmingham in the United Kingdom, the higher the older adults' aerobic fitness level, the lower their probability of experiencing the tip-of-the-tongue state. We've all experienced that phenomenon in which we can't recall and speak a particular word or phrase, despite feeling that "it's right on the tip of my tongue." You know the word you want, but you just can't manage to spit it out.

Laughter Yoga

Believe it or not, exercise can be a laughing matter. Laughter yoga is an exercise program usually done in groups, with participants practicing voluntary, intentional laughter—that often becomes real and contagious laughter. Scientifically, laughter enhances your intake of oxygen-rich air; stimulates your heart, lungs, and muscles; increases the release of endorphins in your brain; and decreases stress. There is much truth in the saying "laughter is the best medicine," believed to have been coined almost ten centuries ago! In *Anatomy of an Illness as Perceived by the Patient*, Norman Cousins recounts how, against all odds, he recovered from a chronic illness by belly laughing for 10 minutes every day and maintaining a positive attitude.[14]

More than 20,000 free social clubs are laughing in 110 countries, with some practicing in senior centers and nursing homes. During the early shutdown of the COVID pandemic, Carolyn enrolled in a laughter yoga class on Zoom, thinking it might keep her spirits up. Here's what she has to say about the experience:

> At first, it felt awkward to force a laugh. But once I got into it, I was laughing for real and felt refreshed and uplifted. It ended up being really fun!

If a more traditional exercise program seems unlikely in your life, try a laughter yoga class. You will connect with others, and you just might discover the power of laughter to instill you with a more positive outlook on life.

Connectedness

The human brain is wired to be social. For decades, studies have shown that nurturing close relationships, if only just a few, and maintaining broader social connections stimulate the brain, strengthen the immune system, reduce the risk of depression, and may slow cognitive decline.

Loneliness, which is a reality for many older adults, can be detrimental to physical and mental well-being. In *Together: The Healing Power of Human Connection in a Sometimes Lonely World*, Dr. Vivek Murthy explains how loneliness shapes the lives of many individuals, especially as they age.[15] According to a 2018 study by the Kaiser Family Foundation, one-fifth of adults in the United States and the United Kingdom reported feeling lonely and lacking meaningful connections with others.[16] Individuals living alone, including almost half of women older than 75, are vulnerable to loneliness.

Fortunately, loneliness can be overcome. *Women Over 70* podcast guest Agnes Loughlin (episode #165) realized at age 60 that she had always been lonely and decided to change that script. She studied various healing modalities and now counsels other women about ways to live in connection. As an advocate for aging women, science journalist Lydia Denworth (episode #63) explains that the feeling of loneliness is your brain's signal that you need to connect. In other words, there is a gap between the social engagement you want and what you currently have. Denworth sees friendship as the best remedy for aging, regardless of whether you live with someone or by yourself. In her book *Friendship*, Denworth offers multiple perspectives on why friendship is essential to well-being during every phase of life.[17] True friendships are long-lasting and stable, make you feel good, and are reciprocal. In essence, friendship is a social relationship that "gets inside your body," having both physical and emotional effects. Friendship also protects you against the stresses of everyday life and hard-hitting life events—it has survival value. Quality matters over quantity: having just one close friend is beneficial. Female friendships have been found to be as, if not more, life sustaining for older women than even a longtime partner.[18]

Let's not overlook the benefits of reciprocal, loving relationships with our pets. The unconditional acceptance and love of a pet can be a tonic for depression, anxiety, loneliness, and social isolation. Indeed, research has found that patients with Alzheimer disease show less verbal aggression and anxiety in the presence of animals. That is why some dementia units have a resident dog or cat. On the home front,

Catherine has loved dogs since her childhood on the farm and has had canine companions nearly all her life. Leo, a Shih Tzu, was a bonding force between Catherine and her daughter during the teenage years. Later, as an empty nester, Catherine enjoyed many years of companionship with her two delightful Bichons, Lucy and Sophie, until each passed from complications of old age.

In *The Awakened Brain*, we learn from researcher Lisa Miller, PhD, that connection can be examined on yet another plane—the spiritual.[19] Using fMRI scans, Miller found that specific areas of the brain were activated when the participants retold a spiritual experience. These narratives were diverse: some were religious services in song or prayer, others retold a spiritual awakening in nature, and yet others recalled transcendence during music and athletic events. Miller could see activation in areas of the brain when a participant had a flash of clarity or sensation of being absorbed by something larger—of going beyond the body and being part of something greater than themselves—an awakened awareness. Whatever pathway to spiritual awakening the participants chose to tell, religious or secular, the same part of the brain was activated. This connection to spirit can be nurtured in many ways. Catherine recalls a significant awakening when she was 19 years old and felt, for the first time, the vastness and power of the Atlantic Ocean. Now, as an adult long-gone from the farm, seeing fields of yellow sunflowers, golden wheat, or green corn arouses vivid memories of playing and working in a multigenerational family. For her, this sense of belonging is a spiritual connection.

Drs. Bredesen and Gupta offer compelling messages of hope that the brain can continually improve and get sharper throughout your life. You can fortify your brain's resilience and overall health through a comprehensive approach that includes exercise, healthy eating, supplements, brain stimulation, close interpersonal relationships, community engagement, and awakened awareness. We are especially inspired by Dr. Miller's conclusion that a spiritual connection is good for the brain.

PATHWAYS TO STIMULATE BRAIN HEALTH

Self-Awareness: What does a healthy brain mean to you? Do you have any concerns about how your brain is functioning?

Self-Compassion: When you notice changes that might be unsettling, be curious about them. Be forgiving of small losses and appreciate new capacities.

Self-Advocacy: It is never too late. What strategies could you use to enliven the health of your brain?

CATHERINE'S PATHWAY

Once I got through brain fog during two long rounds of menopausal symptoms, my brain has functioned quite well. Perhaps I have my mother's genes who, at age 96, has relatively good brain functioning. For years, my mother has urged me to "stop working so hard," especially since my semi-retirement in 2019. Many reminders later—that my projects keep my brain healthy—she may have acquiesced. My brain loves new learning, ever since I was a young girl, waiting impatiently for the book mobile to arrive every 2 weeks at my one-room country schoolhouse. My brain seduces me to take on projects where I can delve into new ideas and material and develop more skills. Sometimes this results in too much of a good thing, but it all keeps me energized.

Sanjay Gupta advises that new pathways in the brain are created when doing or learning something new. Two recent experiences, far outside my normal patterns, I'm sure have created new pathways. Just prior to retiring from DePaul University, I took intensive training in how to design online courses, assuming that I would have plenty of time to practice and be prepared to offer something in the distant future. However, due to the sudden onset of COVID, I had less than 3 weeks to redesign an in-person course for online and offer it via Zoom. For that intimidating task, I had a good deal of support from my college's instructional designer. In subsequent quarters, I pushed ahead on my own to set up and navigate the online learning platform and create an interactive learning community on Zoom. Thankfully, I had extensive experience designing courses so at least I had that foundation to draw on. That was not the case for the podcast, Women Over 70: Aging Reimagined, *that my partner, Gail, and I decided to launch. I seldom listened to podcasts and was uninformed about what creating and running one would involve. Gail and I took a podcast immersion course and sprang into action. During that first year, learning the language, technology, and logistics of podcasting was an enormous stretch.*

I am keen on keeping my brain healthy. As I've discussed in previous chapters, I am paying closer attention to nutrition, exercise, and the signals my body sends out. I am more intentional about seeking spiritual connections, especially through nature.

Part III

Harmonize Your Body, Mind, and Spirit

The focus of the last chapter is on your whole self. As a vital, aging woman, you can nurture your spirit, your self-compassion, and your purpose while pursuing new pathways to holistic health.

Celebrate your life beyond menopause. The years ahead are your opportunity to create your life as you want it. Shape your environment by choosing nourishing relationships with people, food, and nature. Share your knowledge and spirit with others, and stay curious to new possibilities that give life meaning.

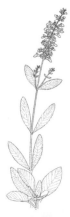

Salvia officinalis (Sage)

DOI: 10.1201/9781003250968-14

12 Nurturing the Mature Woman

A tree with deep intersecting roots, supple yet sturdy trunk, and vibrantly colored leaves on branches reaching forward as new pathways unfold. This image on our book cover symbolizes nourishment, growth, and movement toward what's yet to come. Imagine that this is your tree. It represents the durable foundation of health you have already built for yourself. It invites you to nourish new growth and reach toward new possibilities to enhance your vitality.

Self-nurturing is essential to your health. What do you see when you look at your life as a whole? How mindful are you of your life experiences and intuitive knowing that continue to shape your life? How intentional are you about practicing self-compassion, rebounding from loss, cultivating purpose, and sustaining resilience? These self-nurturing attitudes and behaviors call on your mind, body, and spirit to work together to create new pathways to holistic living.

NURTURING BODY-SPIRIT

Your body affects and is affected by your emotional, mental, and spiritual qualities. Consider this metaphor: *your body is the suitcase for your soul.* We see soul and spirit as intertwined and use the language of spirit and spirituality. We think of *spirit* as the vital force within each of us. Derived from the Latin *spiritus*, it means "soul, courage, vigor, breath." The spirit, then, is the nonphysical part of your vital core. In a holistic sense, and in your unique way, your spiritual health is inextricably connected to your mental, emotional, social, and physical health.

Postmenopause is a passage in life when women are primed to grow spiritually. Many women reveal that their heart opens to connect more profoundly with themselves, others, and the natural world. Tina Turner, the Queen of Rock 'n' Roll, at age 81, speaks to this:

> I don't perform any more . . . I do other things and think any creative endeavor helps to nourish my soul. Whether it's reading, writing, painting, singing, gardening, volunteering or even caring for pets or loved ones.[1]

As Turner is nourishing her soul, she is also nourishing her brain. Lisa Miller, PhD, author of *The Awakened Brain*,[2] might say that Turner exemplifies the brain-spirit connection. Miller's research led her to conclude that a spiritual brain is a healthier brain. She says that with spiritual awakening comes the choice to perceive the world more fully and thus enhance your life. She also notes that the brain responds to spiritual experiences, whether secular or religious.

What spirit or spirituality means to you may change as you age. For some of you, spirituality is tantamount to a particular religion. If you moved away from your

DOI: 10.1201/9781003250968-15

religious upbringing sometime during adulthood, you might be seeking reconnection with and renewal of your faith. Some of you might be exchanging religious dogma for spiritual principles. Those of you with a secular orientation may become more intentional about connecting with a higher power or purpose. You might seek serenity and contentment through meditation or being with the natural world. Another perspective is from the teaching of the Dalai Lama: *"My religion is kindness."* Kindness, to yourself and others, is at the core of spiritual connection and human flourishing.

NURTURING SELF-COMPASSION

For over 20 years, researcher Kristen Neff, PhD, has encouraged women to practice "self-kindness." She portrayed "tender self-compassion" as the voice that assures you it's okay to be present with whatever discomfort or suffering you are experiencing. The voice of tender self-compassion encourages you to observe your thoughts and feelings with an open mind, without trying to suppress, deny, or judge them. Neff now asserts that this form of self-compassion, while necessary, often is not sufficient. In her recent book *Fierce Self-Compassion*,[3] Neff advises women to also exert "fierce self-compassion" to claim what they need and chart a path for putting it into action.

Following is a powerful example of a voice of self-advocacy.

> *At the age of 60, Betsy was full of anger. Her marriage of 30 years suddenly dissolved when her husband left her for another woman. Heartbroken, Betsy recognized that she could not manage on her own. She sought professional counseling and joined a women's support group where she realized she was not alone in her struggles. She also found a local meditation community that helped her let go of pain and anger and develop a more positive outlook. The next couple of years were very challenging, but with community support and a regular meditation practice, Betsy was able to shift her anger about what she had lost to curiosity about what her new life might hold. She learned to cultivate her voice of self-compassion—tenderly and fiercely—which empowered her sense of purpose and resilience.*

Undoubtedly, you can think of numerous life situations when your self-compassion has needed to be both tender and fierce. Let's consider an especially challenging task—the act of forgiveness. Forgiveness involves releasing an expectation that is causing you to suffer. In Betsy's case, she realized that anger about what her life was missing kept her from feeling healthy and at peace with her life. Tara Brach, PhD, psychologist, author, and meditation teacher, points out that "we can't simply will ourselves into forgiving; but we can be willing."[4] That is why the intention to forgive is such a key element in the healing process. It requires an attitude of "letting go" of judgments and attachments about how people and situations should be. Forgiveness is an internal experience that opens up your heart—your spiritual energy—to release lingering pain and generate resilience for well-being.

NURTURING LOSS

The road to aging nearly always involves changes that disrupt our lives in some way. With regard to physical health, for example, breast cancer often requires treatments that can be difficult to tolerate and, while successful, may have unanticipated long-term effects. Complications after a hip replacement might change your expectation of what it feels like to move naturally. Arthritis may also limit mobility. You may need to switch up running for swimming, tennis for pickleball, or floor yoga for chair yoga. Physical changes such as these are what Pauline Boss, PhD, calls "ambiguous loss."[5] These kinds of changes are not debilitating enough to have an official label or a ritual to acknowledge the change. Having a name for what you are feeling—ambiguous loss—can help you adjust to new realities.

Emotional health is equally important or perhaps even more so than physical health. By the postmenopausal time of life, many of you are all too familiar with experiencing the loss of loved ones. You might lose family members, adult children, friends, and pets. Death of one's life partner can be particularly devastating. The person with whom you connected most deeply is gone; responsibilities once shared are now on your shoulders; relationship dynamics may change with friends and family members; finances need to be managed differently. You may need to decide where you will live in the future.

While anticipating the future is important, it is not the first priority. Whether someone's death is anticipated or unexpected, grief is inevitable and natural, and the grieving process is absolutely necessary. In *Warrior Mother: A Memoir of Fierce Love, Unbearable Loss, and Rituals That Heal*,[6] Sheila Collins shares lessons learned after the deaths of her two children. During her interview on the podcast *Women Over 70: Aging Reimagined* (episode #99), Sheila describes the oscillating nature of grief. She uses the metaphor of the surf rising and falling with the tides. At times it's an easy rhythm of the calm sea, while at other times it calls on all your strength to withstand the intensity and frequency of the waves. Riding the waves of grief requires resilience to move through the difficulties and, over time, bounce back with new attitudes and purpose. In *Wise Aging: Living With Joy, Resilience and Spirit*,[7] Cowan and Thal affirm that this is possible.

> *In challenging times, we discover our courage and resilience; we learn that we can bear sadness; we learn that we can appreciate love and beauty in the midst of loss. Often this surprises us . . . that we have reaped benefit from an occurrence that we judge unfair or even tragic.*[8]

How is this possible? Mary-Frances O'Connor, PhD, explains that grieving involves a tough kind of learning.[9] Fortunately, your brain is a learning organism; as such, you come to learn that your loved one no longer exists in the dimensions you once knew. "We find new ways to express our continuing bonds transforming what 'close' looks like because our loved one remains in the epigenetics of our DNA and in our memories." We learn how to adapt to the loss of being together and, over time, to focus on the process of reconstructing a meaningful life.

NURTURING PURPOSE

Purpose, of course, does not only emanate from adjusting to hardships. It comes in many forms, under different circumstances, and with different meanings. We like the translation of purpose from the Japanese word *ikigai:* a sense of well-being from being alive. People with purpose are also known to be more resilient, which means they have the capacity to adapt and persist under difficult circumstances. Tara Brach explains that the seeds of purpose are already within you and can always be culti-vated. Having purpose for some women involves championing women's rights, while for others it may focus on relationships with family and friends. Yet others nurture their inner selves through reading, writing, or being in nature. Your sense of purpose is unique to you and need not be compared with that of others.

Mounting evidence from large-scale studies reveals how pursuing a purpose can make a person happier and healthier—and even lengthen their life span. Dr. Robert Butler and collaborators studied the correlation between having a sense of purpose and longevity. It is clear that individuals who express a clear goal in life—something to get up for in the morning, something that makes a difference—live longer and are sharper than those who do not pursue a purpose.

As We Close

We hope this book has helped you gain deeper insight into how you know yourself and more confidence in advocating for yourself. We have encouraged you to explore a range of holistic options, to work toward collaborative relationships with your prac-titioners, and to establish an adaptable web of wellness. We trust that rewarding discoveries await you as you pursue new pathways to holistic living. We are confident that you will flourish as you move through your postmenopausal years.

We now invite you, in the spirit of holistic health, to join us in making an emboldened declaration:

As postmenopausal women, we expect to be seen, heard, and respected. We assume responsibility to advocate for the care we need. With empowered voices, we lay claim to holistic integrative health approaches that enable us to remain vital and engaged in life with purpose and resilience.

References

INTRODUCTION

1. Vincent GK, Velkoff VA. *The Next Four Decades, the Older Population in the United States: 2010 to 2050, Current Population Reports*. US Census Bureau; 2010:25–1138.
2. Palmore E. Ageism comes of age. *J Gerontol B Psychol Sci Soc Sci*. 2015;70(6):873–875.
3. Gullette MM. *Ending Ageism, or How Not to Shoot Old People*. Rutgers University Press; 2017.

CHAPTER 1

1. Pizzorno J. How to cure the sick health care system: an open letter to President Trump from leaders in functional/integrative/natural health and medicine. *Integr Med*. 2017;16(1):8–11.

CHAPTER 2

1. Immordino-Yang MH. *Emotions, Learning, and the Brain: Exploring the Educational Implications of Affective Neuroscience*. W.W. Norton & Company; 2015.
2. Tolle E. *The Power of Now: A Guide to Spiritual Enlightenment*. Namaste; 1999.
3. Reeves P. *Women's Intuition: Unlocking the Wisdom of the Body*. Conari Press; 1999:252.
4. Belenky M, Clinchy B, Goldberger N, et al. *Women's Ways of Knowing: The Development of Self, Voice, and Mind*. Basic Books; 1996.

CHAPTER 3

1. Gawande A. *Being Mortal: Medicine and What Matters in the End*. Metropolitan Books; 2014:304.
2. Kegan R, Lahey LL. *Immunity to Change: How to Overcome It and Unlock Potential in Yourself and Your Organization*. Harvard Business School Press; 2009:340.

CHAPTER 4

1. Smith T, Sahni S, Thacker HL. Postmenopausal hormone therapy-local and systemic: a pharmacologic perspective. *J Clin Pharmacol*. 2020;60(Suppl 2):S74–S85.
2. Boston Women's Health Collective. *Our Bodies, Ourselves*. New England Free Press; 1971.
3. Murray MT. *Menopause: You Can Benefit from Diet, Vitamins, Minerals, Herbs, Exercise, and Other Natural Methods*. Getting Well Naturally; 1994.
4. Wright JM. *Natural Hormones Replacement for Women Over 45*. Smart Publications; 1997.
5. Lee J. *What Your Doctor May Not Tell You About Menopause*. Grand Central Publishing; 1996.
6. Cagnacci A, Venier M. The controversial history of hormone replacement therapy. *Medicina (Kaunas)*. 2019;55(9):602.

7. Chlebowski RT, Anderson GL, Aragaki AK, et al. Association of menopausal hormone therapy with breast cancer incidence and mortality during long-term follow-up of the Women's Health Initiative randomized clinical trials. *JAMA*. 2020;324(4):369–380.

8. Kling JM, MacLaughlin KL, Schnatz PF, et al. Menopause management knowledge in postgraduate family medicine, internal medicine, and obstetrics and gynecology residents: a cross-sectional survey. *Mayo Clin Proc*. 2019;94(2):242–253.

9. Panel TNHTPSA. The 2017 hormone therapy position statement of the North American Menopause Society. *Menopause*. 2017;24(7):728–753.

10. Brown DE, Sievert LL, Morrison LA, et al. Do Japanese American women really have fewer hot flashes than European Americans? The Hilo Women's Health Study. *Menopause*. 2009;16(5):870–876.

11. Barnard N. The women's study for the alleviation of vasomotor symptoms (WAVS): a randomized, controlled trial of a plant-based diet and whole soybeans for postmenopausal women. *Menopause*. 2021;28(10):1150–1156.

12. Baudry J, Assmann KE, Touvier M, et al. Association of frequency of organic food consumption with cancer risk: findings from the NutriNet-santé prospective cohort study. *JAMA Intern Med*. 2018;178(12):1597–1606.

13. Meehan M, Penckofer S. The role of vitamin D in the aging adult. *J Aging Gerontol*. 2014;2(2):60–71.

14. Shah K, Varna VP, Pandya A, et al. Low vitamin D levels and prognosis in a COVID-19 paediatric population: a systematic review. *QJM*. 2021;114(7):447–453.

15. CRN. Dietary Supplement Usage Increases, Says New Survey, 2017. https://www.crnusa.org/newsroom/dietary-supplement-usage-increases-says-new-survey

16. Chiu HY, Pan CH, Shyu YK, et al. Effects of acupuncture on menopause-related symptoms and quality of life in women in natural menopause: a meta-analysis of randomized controlled trials. *Menopause*. 2015;22(2):234–244.

CHAPTER 5

1. University of Michigan. *National Poll on Healthy Aging*. University of Michigan, May 2018.

2. Paine EA, Umberson D, Reczek C. Sex in midlife: women's sexual experiences in lesbian and straight marriages. *J Marriage Fam*. 2019;81(1):7–23.

3. Lindau ST, Schumm LP, Laumann EO, et al. A study of sexuality and health among older adults in the United States. *N Engl J Med*. 2007;357:762–774.

4. Granville L, Pregler J. Women's sexual health and aging. *J Am Geriatr Soc*. 2018;66(3):595–601.

5. Kahn Ladas A, Whipple B, Perry JD. *The G Spot: And Other Discoveries About Human Sexuality*. Holt Paperbacks; First Owl Book Edition; 2005.

6. Price J. *The Ultimate Guide to Sex After Fifty: How to Maintain—or Regain—a Spicy, Satisfying Sex Life*. Cleis Press; 2015.

7. Bhupathiraju SN, Grodstein F, Stampfer MJ, et al. Vaginal estrogen use and chronic disease risk in the nurses' health study. *Menopause*. 2018;26(6):603–610.

8. Khamba B, Aucoin M, Lytle M, et al. Efficacy of acupuncture treatment of sexual dysfunction secondary to antidepressants. *J Altern Complement Med*. 2013;19(11):862–869.

CHAPTER 6

1. El Khoudary SR, Greendale G, Crawford SL, et al. The menopause transition and women's health at midlife: a progress report from the study of women's health across the nation (SWAN). *Menopause*. 2019;26(10):1213–1227.

2. Walker M. *Why We Sleep: Unlocking the Power of Sleep and Dreams*. Penguin Random House; 2017.
3. Gupta S. *Keep Sharp: Build a Better Brain at Any Age*. Simon & Schuster; 2021.
4. Emmons H. *Chemistry of Joy*. Fireside; 2005.
5. Emmons H. *Chemistry of Calm*. Simon & Schuster; 2010.
6. Faydalı S, Çetinkaya F. The effect of aromatherapy on sleep quality of elderly people residing in a nursing home. *Holist Nurs Pract*. 2018;32(1):8–16.

CHAPTER 7

1. Hantsoo L, Epperson CN. Anxiety disorders among women: a female lifespan approach. *Focus (Am Psychiatr Publ)*. 2017;15(2):162–172.
2. Wehrwein P. Astounding increase in antidepressant use by Americans. *Harvard Health Blog*. https://www.health.harvard.edu/blog/astounding-increase-in-antidepressant-use-by-americans-201110203624
3. Tolle E. *The Power of Now: A Guide to Spiritual Enlightenment*. Namaste; 1999.
4. World Health Organization. *Doing What Matters in Times of Stress: An Illustrated Guide*. 2020. https://www.who.int/publications/i/item/9789240003927
5. Das R. *Be Here Now*. Harmony/Rodale; 1971.
6. Chödrön P, Boucher S. *Taking the Leap: Freeing Ourselves from Old Habits and Fears*. Shambhala Publications, Inc.; 2009.
7. Neston J. *Breath: The New Science of a Lost Art*. Riverhead Books; 2020.
8. Baltzell J. *Why Meditation Works*. Polair Publishing; 2006.
9. Kabat-Zinn J. *Wherever You Go There You Are*. Hyperion; 1994.
10. Auster S. *Sound Bath: Meditate, Heal and Connect Through Listening*. S&S/Simon Element; 2019.
11. Hackenmiller SB. *The Outdoor Adventurer's Guide to Forest Bathing*. Falcon Guides; 2019.
12. Mirman J. *Demystifying Homeopathy: A Concise Guide to Homeopathic Medicine*. New Hope Publishers; 2009.

CHAPTER 8

1. Bland J. *The 20-Day Rejuvenation Diet Program*. McGraw Hill; 1999.
2. Wahls T. *The Wahls Protocol: A Radical New Way to Treat All Chronic Autoimmune Conditions Using Paleo Principles*. Avery; 2014.
3. Teitelbaum J. *From Fatigue to Fantastic: A Clinically Proven Program to Regain Vibrant Health and Overcome Chronic Fatigue*. Avery; 2020.
4. Vasquez A, MacDonald Baker S, Bennett P, et al. *Textbook of Functional Medicine*. Institute for Functional Medicine; 2010.
5. Pacini S, Fiore MG, Magherini S, et al. Could cadmium be responsible for some of the neurological signs and symptoms of myalgic encephalomyelitis/chronic fatigue syndrome. *Med Hypotheses*. 2012;79(3):403–407.

CHAPTER 9

1. Kapoor E, Collazo-Clavell ML, et al. Weight gain in women at midlife: a concise review of the pathophysiology and strategies for management. *Mayo Clin Proc*. 2017;92(10):1552–1558.
2. Mangweth-Matzek B, Rupp CI, Hausmann A, et al. Never too old for eating disorders or body dissatisfaction: a community study of elderly women. *Int J Eat Disord*. 2006;39(7):583–586.

3. Gagne DA, Von Holle A, Brownley KA, et al. Eating disorder symptoms and weight and shape concerns in a large web-based convenience sample of women ages 50 and above: results of the gender and body image (GABI) study. *Int J Eat Disord.* 2012;45(7):832–844.
4. Dudrick S. Older clients and eating disorders. *Today's Dietitian.* 2014;15(11):44.
5. CDC. Center for Disease Control, Obesity Rates. https://www.cdc.gov/obesity/data/adult.html
6. World Health Organization: Obesity & Overweight. https://www.who.int/news-room/fact-sheet/detail/obesity-and-overweight
7. Ellulu MS, Patimah I, Khaza'ai H, et al. Obesity and inflammation: the linking mechanism and the complications. *Arch Med Sci.* 2017;13(4):851–863.
8. Mann T. *Secrets from the Eating Lab.* Harper Collins; 2015.
9. Sindhu K, Reddy P. Resident Physicians; Weight Shaming. *Think Newsletter.* Aug 24, 2019.
10. Pont SJ, Puhl R, Cook SR, et al. Stigma experienced by children and adolescents with obesity. *Pediatrics.* 2017;140(6):e20173034.
11. D'Adamo P. *Eat Right 4 Your Type.* Penguin Random House; 1996.
12. Willis B, Shanmugam R, Southerland J, et al. Food allergen elimination for obesity reduction; a longitudinal, case-control trial. *Brit J Gastroenterol.* 2020;2(4):199–203.
13. Pollan M. *Food Rules: An Eater's Manual.* Penguin Books; 2009:140.
14. Menzel J, Jabakhanji A, Biemann R, et al. Systematic review and meta-analysis of the associations of vegan and vegetarian diets with inflammatory biomarkers. *Sci Rep.* 2020;10(1):21736.
15. Kahleova H, Rembert E, Alwarith J, et al. Effects of a low-fat vegan diet on gut microbiota in overweight individuals and relationships with body weight, body composition, and insulin sensitivity: a randomized clinical trial. *Nutrients.* 2020;12(10):2917.
16. Lee IM, Djoussé L, Sesso HD, et al. Physical activity and weight gain prevention. *JAMA.* 2010;303(12):1173–1179.
17. O'Mara S. *In Praise of Walking: A New Scientific Exploration.* W.W. Norton & Company; 2021.

CHAPTER 10

1. Bone Health and Osteoporosis Foundation. What Women Need to Know. https://www.bonehealthandosteoporosis.org/preventing-fractures/general-facts/what-women-need-to-know/
2. Iarocci T. Preventing an Epidemic of New Osteoporotic Fractures in America. https://expertperspectives.com/Osteoporosis/Osteoporosis/preventing-an-epidemic-of-new-osteoporotic-fractures-in-america
3. LeBlanc KE, Muncie HL Jr, LeBlanc LL. Hip fracture: diagnosis, treatment, and secondary prevention. *Am Fam Physician.* 2014;89(12):945–951.
4. NAMS Position Statement. Management of osteoporosis in postmenopausal women: the 2021 position statement of the North American Menopause Society. *Menopause.* 2021;28(9):973–997.
5. Wallace T, Jun S, Zou P, et al. Dairy intake is not associated with improvements in bone mineral density or risk of fractures across the menopause transition: data from the Study of Women's Health Across the Nation. *Menopause.* 2020;27(8):879–886.
6. Fishman L, Saltonstall E. *Yoga for Osteoporosis: The Complete Guide.* W.W. Norton & Company; 2010.

CHAPTER 11

1. Lunden J. *Why Did I Come Into This Room?: A Candid Conversation About Aging.* Forefront Books; 2020.
2. World Health Organization. Dementia. Sept 2021. https://www.who.int/news-room/fact-sheets/detail/dementia
3. Mosconi L. *The XX Brain.* Penguin Random House; 2020.
4. Mehegan L, Rainville C, Skufca L. 2017 Brain health and nutrition survey. *Family Med News.* Jan 2018.
5. Doidge N. *The Brain That Changes Itself.* Penguin Publishing Group; 2007.
6. Gupta S. *Keep Sharp: Build a Better Brain at Any Age.* Simon & Schuster; 2021.
7. Baker L. Multi-Domain Lifestyle Interventions to Prevent Cognitive Decline and Dementia. Presented at the 2021 Dementia Prevention Conference, Nov 19, 2021.
8. Kivipelto M, Mangialasche F, Snyder HM, et al. World-wide FINGERS network: a global approach to risk reduction and prevention of dementia. *Alzheimers Dement.* 2020;16(7):1078–1094.
9. Morris MC, Tangney CC, Wang Y, et al. MIND diet associated with reduced incidence of Alzheimer's disease. *Alzheimers Dement.* 2015;11(9):1007–1014.
10. Buettner D. *The Blue Zones: Lessons for Living Longer from the People Who've Lived the Longest.* National Geographic; 2008.
11. Bredesen D. *The End of Alzheimer's: The First Program to Prevent and Reserve Cognitive Decline.* Penguin Random House; 2007.
12. Littlejohns TJ, Henley WE, Lang IA, et al. Vitamin D and the risk of dementia and Alzheimer disease. *Neurology.* 2014;83(10):920–928.
13. Perlmutter D. *The Brain Maker: The Power of Gut Microbes to Heal and Protect Your Brain for Life.* Little, Brown Spark; 2015.
14. Cousins N. *Anatomy of an Illness: As Perceived by the Patient: Reflections on Healing and Regeneration.* W.W. Norton & Company, Inc.; 2016.
15. Murthy V. *Together: The Healing Power of Human Connection in a Sometimes Lonely World.* Harper Wave; 2020.
16. DiJulio B, Hamel L, Muñana C, et al. *Loneliness and Social Isolation in the United States, the United Kingdom, and Japan: An International Survey.* August 2018.
17. Denworth L. *Friendship: The Evolution, Biology, and Extraordinary Power of Life's Fundamental Bond.* W.W. Norton & Company; 2020.
18. Fuller-Iglesias HR, Webster NJ, Antonucci TC. Adult family relationships in the context of friendship. *Res Hum Dev.* 2013;10(2):184–203.
19. Miller L. *The Awakened Brain: The New Science of Spirituality and Our Quest for an Inspired Life.* Random House; 2021.

CHAPTER 12

1. Nash A. *Tina Turner's Steps to Happiness.* AARP; Dec 9, 2020.
2. Miller L. *The Awakened Brain: The New Science of Spirituality and Our Quest for an Inspired Life.* Random House; 2021.
3. Neff K. *Fierce Self-Compassion: How Women Can Harness Kindness to Speak Up, Claim Their Power, and Thrive.* HarperCollins; 2021.
4. Brach T. Resources on Forgiveness. https://www.tarabrach.com/forgiveness/
5. Boss P. *Ambiguous Loss: Learning to Live with Unresolved Grief.* Harvard University Press; 2000.

6. Collins S. *Warrior Mother: A Memoir of Fierce Love, Unbearable Loss, and Rituals That Heal.* She Writes Press; 2013.
7. Cowan R, Thal L. *Wise Aging: Living With Joy, Resilience and Spirit.* Behrman House Publishing; 2015.
8. Jonas W. *How Healing Works: Get Well and Stay Well Using Your Hidden Power to Heal.* Lorena Jones Books, Penguin Random House; 2018.
9. O'Connor MF. *The Grieving Brain: The Surprising Science of How We Learn from Love and Loss.* Harper One; 2022.

Acknowledgments

We are blessed with a network of colleagues, family, and friends who have supported the germination and completion of this book. Linda Gesler, our friend for 50 years, has cheered us on since the inception of this undertaking, offering candid feedback during our writing retreats at Carolyn's second home on Isla Mujeres. Linda's dogged search for a publisher led us to CRC Press/Taylor and Francis Group and Senior Editor Randy Brehm, who has been superbly open to our ideas and responsive to our requests. Positive reviews of our book proposal by Bill Manahan, MD, and Kathleen Taylor, PhD, led to the contract signing.

Several people were instrumental in shaping the book's content and architecture. Early contributors were authors and professional editors, Ellen Sue Stern and Barbara Mirel, PhD. Ellen influenced our emphasis on the voice of self-advocacy, and Barbara advised us on creating structural consistency. Miriam Must offered editing on many chapters; her sharp questioning about voice in Part II prompted inclusion of Catherine's Pathways. Karen Marienau, MD, author and editor, bettered the whole manuscript with her medical knowledge and sharp editing eye. Bobbi Krippner took on the job of entering references into EndNote. Then we hit the jackpot with Susan Aiello, DVM, ELS, who became our professional editor for everything—from the overarching framework to the extensive content to all the gritty details involved in readying the manuscript for the publisher. We are extremely grateful to Susan for her enthusiastic support, for her direct and invaluable feedback, and for making our voices sound like us, only better.

In pursuit of a title, we peppered conversations with many people about their reaction to various possibilities; we appreciate their input. Special thanks to Larry Strenge, who chimed in "Why not call it *Beyond Menopause*?" and to Gail Zelitzky for analyzing headlines that led to "New Pathways to Holistic Health."

A good book must have a captivating cover. Reaching far back into our network, we relocated Kathleen Marie Garness, a juried and award-winning artist whose botanical renderings grace the Smithsonian and other prestigious venues. We are enthralled with her illustrations on the cover and the introductory pages to each of the three parts. We thank Christopher Nelson, professional photographer, for agreeing to shoot at Carolyn's home on the island, working effectively around tight spaces, shifting light and wind and nervous subjects.

From Catherine: I credit my collaborators on other projects for contributing a rich knowledge base about women, aging, and brain science. Karla Klinger first got me interested in older women through our 10-year study on "*Vital Women Over 70.*" Kathleen Taylor has been my companion into neuroscience and adult learning and my mentor on writing in a nonacademic style. Through Women Over 70, LLC, my co-host, Gail Zelitzky, and I are showing the world that older women are vitally engaged in life. Thanks to each of them for supporting me when *Beyond Menopause* required priority. I appreciate ongoing encouragement from other author friends,

Pamela Meyer, PhD, and James Cogan. My personal trainer, Janice Enloe, keeps me moving. Ever since I first mentioned this project, my sister Karen has offered much encouragement. Anna Roth, my daughter, motivates me to live beyond a life of the mind. She offers loving support and is proud of her mom.

From Carolyn: Many people and places have supported my journey in holistic, integrative medicine. Neil Nathan, MD, was an early mentor and became a trusted colleague. Bill Manahan, MD, has been my prominent person in all things holistic for some 30 years. The Women's Health Specialists Clinic at the University of Minnesota provided me the space to practice integrative medicine. Special thanks to my visionary colleagues Diana Drake, Anne Coetzee, and Carrie Terrell. Deep appreciation to the Department of Family Medicine and Dr. James Pacala for granting me a sabbatical to begin the work on this book. My dear friends on the island Greta Shorey Kramer, MD, and Margo Chapman Kendall helped lighten the mood by sharing enjoyable meals and laughing at my quirky poems. I thank my daughter, Erica, and her family for always welcoming me with loving, open arms. Last, but not least, I say thank you to my husband and soul mate, Brad Beneke, for being by my side for the past 40+ years.

———

We are both grateful to the women in Carolyn's clinical practice and in Catherine's higher learning setting, and to all the other women we know, for giving us insights into the extraordinary lives of postmenopausal women. And we are grateful for our home-away-from-home, Isla Mujeres, for providing respite and inspiration.

Carolyn Torkelson, MD
Catherine Marienau, PhD

Index